AUGSBURG COLLEGE
Department of Nursing

NURSING CARE OF THE ELDERLY

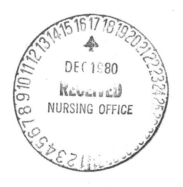

NURSING CARE OF THE ELDERLY

Helen I. Weber

RESTON PUBLISHING COMPANY, INC.
A Prentice-Hall Company
Reston, Virginia

Library of Congress Cataloging in Publication Data

Weber, Helen I
  Nursing care of the elderly.

  Includes bibliographies and index.
  1. Geriatric nursing. I. Title.
  [DNLM: 1. Geriatric nursing.   WY152 W374m]
  RC954.W32   610.73'65   80-11053
  ISBN 0-8359-5035-2

© 1980 by Reston Publishing Company, Inc.
A Prentice-Hall Company
Reston, Virginia 22090

10 9 8 7 6 5 4 3 2 1

Printed in the United States of America

TO HATTIE AND KATE,
TWO GALLANT MOTHERS IN
THEIR 80TH AND 90TH YEARS

Contents

Preface

This book has been written primarily for the practical/vocational student nurse, although other nursing personnel may find it useful.

For convenience, "he" has been used to describe most patients, "she" to describe the nurse. This does not indicate that the author is not aware of the importance of women in every area of life, nor that she is unaware of the valuable contributions of the male nurse.

The services of the LPN/LVN in the care of the elderly adult are invaluable. The need for more graduates increases each year, as do the responsibilities they are expected to fulfill.

Nursing Care of the Elderly Adult was written to help the student nurse understand some of the problems the elderly patient faces before he comes to a nursing home. Not every aspect of institutionalized care is covered: it is assumed that the student is enrolled in classes that teach basic nursing care, anatomy, nutrition, and other necessary subjects. Only those areas that have been identified as common problems in the care of the elderly have been included.

The care of the elderly person deserves to be in the hands of those who are determined that it be positive, where nurses resolve that their care will give the patient as many choices as are possible, where regimentation is unknown, where love and touching are lavish, and where the reminiscences and accomplishments of the patient's past are cherished as part of our common heritage.

Nurses are citizens also, and in addition to giving excellent care, they must concern themselves with the machinations of government agencies in their communities and throughout the nation in the attempt to provide care for the aged. The concerned citizen-nurse must speak out and work for change. Her expertise far surpasses that of many of the planners of health programs, and must be heard.

Whether or not the nursing student ever cares for the elderly person in a long-term care facility, it is the author's hope that in addition to making her aware of some of the problems of the elderly, she will also begin to think of her own mortality and plan her life so that her later years will be active and happy.

I wish to express my gratitude to those who assisted me in writing this book:

- To Dortha McCarthy and all of her staff at Southwestern Oregon Community College;
- To Doris Wilson, RN, friend and photographer, for the beautiful studies of the elderly;
- To the Sisters of Mercy and the staff of St. Catherines' Residence and Nursing Home of North Bend, Oregon;
- To the J. T. Posey Company for photographs;
- To my reviewers;
- To Patricia Yeager, a new friend and fine typist;
- To Dave Culverwell, my editor, for kind words and encouragement;
- To my husband, who encouraged me, cracked his whip, and never complained about the time I spent in writing.

HELEN I. WEBER

NURSING CARE OF THE ELDERLY

chapter 1

Introduction to Care of the Elderly Adult

OBJECTIVES

After studying this unit, the student will be able to:

1. Identify some changes in our society that have occurred since 1900 that have led to problems for elderly adults.

2. Discuss some of the reasons for the large proportions of elderly people in our total population.

3. Identify why the responsibilities of a Licensed Practical Nurse are greater in a long-term care facility.

4. Define philosophy of care, policies, procedures, and objectives of a long-term care facility.

5. Define or describe the differences between institutional care, home care, home health care, and homemakers.

THE STUDY OF PROBLEMS OF THE AGED

Many aspects of our everyday life are accepted as "normal," until they become problems that affect the lives of a number of citizens or communities. Air pollution, clean water, wildlife preservation, energy shortages and many other facets of our lives are now studied closely because they present problems that affect our society. In the early years of the century, little was done or thought about these man-made problems.

The study of the aged came about because of the rapidly increased number of older adults in our society and the increasing difficulties they have had in coping with a multitude of problems in their daily lives. These problems have been fostered by the tremendous growth in our population and the change from a predominately rural population to an urban one. In less than a century, our way of life has changed from a rural, horse-drawn culture to an urban, jet-oriented culture that has seen a man walking on the moon: these changes have been particularly difficult for the elderly adult to adapt to.

What brought about this explosion of elderly adults in our society? The total number of births in the last 100 years has greatly increased, and modern medicine, public health knowledge, and better nutrition have increased the number of surviving infants. Thus, more persons survive to 65 years and beyond. The population of the United States was also greatly increased in the late nineteenth and early twentieth centuries by the arrival of immigrants from around the world. These persons are now part of the elderly population.

Table 1-1 shows the increasing 65+ population. As life expectancies have increased, the proportion of the elderly to the entire population has also increased and will continue to do so. One might

3

TABLE 1-1
The Percentage of Total Population, Age 65 and Over in the United States for Selected Years

	1900	1939	1940	1950	1960	1970	2000 (projected)
Percentage age 65 and over	4.0	5.4	6.8	8.1	9.2	9.6	11.1

Source: U.S. Bureau of Census

anticipate that unless current problems are solved, they, too, will continue to increase.

In 1900, only 40 percent of the population lived in cities. In 1960, 70 percent were city dwellers, and it is estimated that by the year 2000, 90 percent will live in metropolitan areas. In 1960, 70 percent of the 65+ population lived in cities, the same percentage as the total population. More elderly persons, however, lived in towns of under 10,000.

Many persons have written about "the good old days" when several generations of a family lived in one house. This may not have been by choice, but due primarily to the fact that only one dwelling place was financially feasible or available, and several wage earners were necessary to support the group. As wages increased and more housing was available, one-family homes became prevalent, and the older family members no longer lived with nor had the support of a large group of family members. Increased labor-saving devices and new child-rearing practices also reduced the usefulness of the older family members.

In a predominately industrial society such as ours, all members of the work force must be kept employed to assure the economic stability of the country. With increasing numbers of people in the work force as the population grows, and with increased mechanization requiring fewer persons, measures must be taken to prevent an overabundance of workers. Overabundance results in widespread unemployment and all of the problems resulting from this decline. Since the 1900s, the level of education has gradually risen from grammar school or less to high school and college completion. The total number of workers is loosely regulated by this increase in the number of years a person is kept out of the labor market. In addition, by limiting the number of years one may work, further regulation of the job market is achieved. In a relatively short period of time the number of years one may work changed from a lifetime of labor to 65 years. Mandatory retirement has now been largely revoked, with no statistics yet available to demonstrate results. In the past, thousands of workers were retired with fixed incomes, with little understanding or preparation for this drastic change in their lives.

After World War II, which imposed changes on almost every aspect of American life, a withdrawal of society from the elderly adult population occurred. Increased emphasis on the worth, wisdom, and education of the young brought about stereotyping of the older citizen that was largely negative. The elderly adults were on their own—at a time in their lives when income and savings did not keep up with rising costs, when chronic disease and loss of physical strength and endurance occurred, and when death of contemporaries and loss of usefulness and self-esteem was felt.

These facts are all part of the forces that have resulted in the sad plight of the elderly adult in this last quarter of the century. Nurses need to see and understand the problems of aging on a wider scale than simply the physical, disease-oriented care of the patient who happens to be elderly. We are part of a total community, and what affects it affects our physical and mental health, our finances, our religion, and our social practices. As nurses become more knowledgeable about the elderly, they can become, as informed citizens, better advocates of the elderly in the community and in the nation. They can also be more aware of what constitutes good care and therefore demand a high standard of performance from themselves and from all members of the health team.

Definitions of Terms

In many fields of study, the student is faced with a new vocabulary that describes the function, attitudes, and principles of the new subject. So it is with the study of the elderly, *gerontology*, which is derived from the Greek, *geros*, the study of old men. *Geriatrics*, the treatment of the elderly, originally referred to the medical treatment of the elderly; at present, however, the definition has been expanded to include the treatment of social, psychological, and recreational needs of the aged.

The normal loss of functional ability during the later years of life is called *senescence*. Senescence may be defined as the process of aging. The individual may not be very concerned about these changes, as they occur gradually, and people learn to adapt to them in different ways. The process is different with each individual, regardless of his age.

The elderly adult in our society bears many titles—old, elderly, oldster, aged, aging, Golden-Ager, Senior Citizen, Pensioner, Retiree, Older American, 65+, and others. Each title is probably distasteful to some segment of the elderly population, as each one tends to stereotype a group of very individual people. We have elected to use "elderly adult" as a descriptive title, aware that it will not meet universal approval, nor accurately describe each individual.

When is one old? In the past we could legally define it as when one reached the 65th year. However, now that retirement requirements have been modified, it is no longer a legal definition. Perhaps the best definition of "old" is when the individual says he is old.

The word *senile* occurs frequently when people discuss aging and seems to be used as a synonym for it. *Senile* means "pertaining to old age" (Dorland's, Tabor's). *Senility* is defined as the "physical and mental deterioration or infirmities of old age" (Dorland's). *Senile* and *senility* tend to be used incorrectly in a derogatory sense to indicate mental incompetence, rather than to describe normal changes of the aging process. *Senility* has probably been used as a synonym for chronic brain syndrome or senile psychosis, in which true behavioral changes are present, as discussed in Chapter 3.

This text will combine both gerontology and geriatrics, attempting to bring material pertinent to both disciplines to the student nurse as she endeavors to give comprehensive care to the older adult.

Attitudes about Geriatric Nursing

Surveys have demonstrated that nurses prefer to care for patients other than the elderly (Campbell, 1971). In one survey, it was found that both nursing students and interns believed that the majority of elderly people lived in nursing homes (Committee on Aging, 1977). This would indicate a belief that most elderly were disabled, sick, and unable to care for themselves.

The attitude of our general society toward the aged influences many nurses in their negative perceptions of old age. Many feel that there is no challenge in geriatrics because the results can only be in one direction. *Attitudes* are learned feelings that result from family, background, education, and society. The attitudes learned at present concerning aging are largely negative, and this is wasteful to our society and damaging to the elderly adult. The stigma that Americans and other societies have attached to old age causes elderly persons to be shunned and rejected. In our rejection of the elderly as equal partners in life, we have lost some of the early principles of our country concerning the worth of each individual citizen. We discount precious first-hand historians and the experiences of those who were leaders and doers of yesterday.

With our societal emphasis on youth and beauty, which is constantly beamed at us through the various media, many people feel that only the young are alert, independent, functioning members of society. Nursing instructors, in some instances, have, by their own prejudices, promulgated the feeling to students that geriatrics is not as worthy of their efforts or as demanding of their skills as is nursing in the specialty areas. When all elderly adults are portrayed as smelly, senile, cantankerous, and slow, it is difficult for the nurse to see her patient as an individual with specific care needs.

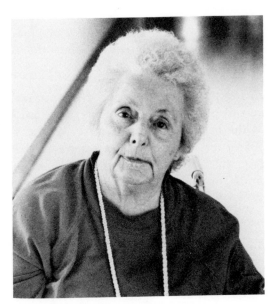

Photographer: Doris Wilson, RN
Model: Minette Walter

Age has a beauty of its own.

If all elderly people in an institution are categorized alike, the tendency is for them to conform and to behave according to the expectations of the care givers. Thus, dependency and unacceptable behavior may become a norm. Self-esteem is lowered or destroyed, and life quickly loses interest and meaning.

The nursing care of the elderly in long-term care facilities is less technical than that in acute care centers, because of the less acute health status and simpler treatment regimes prescribed for the patient. In no other area of nursing are observational skills more important, as physical changes are more covert and the interactions of mental and physical problems more subtle in the elderly adult. The nurse working with the aged adult will have an unprecedented opportunity for use of her interpersonal skills. The sharing of thoughts, ideas, and feelings, as well as listening and caring, are necessary to counteract the patient's feelings of disorientation and loss of self-esteem.

The opportunity for use of self, when no techniques, drugs, nor physician's knowledge will help, makes geriatric nursing both challenging and rewarding. To make the patient's remaining years active, happy, and secure is as challenging as any task within the human realm.

In summarizing thoughts about attitudes, perhaps Halleck (1968), in speaking of our need to relate to the old people in our society, says it best:

> In drifting into a youth-oriented culture we have ignored the teachings of philosophers who have since the time of Plato emphasized the need to revere maturity. We are often told that our youth are our future. Yet, unless we can create a world which offers the possibility of aging with grace, honor and meaningfulness, no one can look forward to the future.

THE ROLE OF THE PRACTICAL NURSE IN CARING FOR THE ELDERLY ADULT

The responsibility for the care of the elderly, and particularly the care of the sick elderly, is one shared by the government (federal and state), the health professions, and each individual. In some instances, the responsibility is financial, in others it is regulatory, but most important is our individual moral responsibility toward the elderly adult. Old model machines can be discarded. Old people cannot—must not—be treated in this manner. Retirement from the work force does not mean that the person does not contribute to society. If he does not visibly contribute, he is no less a human, and no less deserving of our respect and care.

The technology and the financial ability to provide care for the aged is readily available in the United States. The issue is primarily one of priorities. A portion of the individual's moral responsibility may be to act as an advocate for the elderly. Politically, the persons in nursing homes and their families are not active nor powerful, although organizations such as the Grey Panthers are beginning to effect some changes. If we are convinced of our duty, we must act positively in supporting the legislation necessary for the proper care for our elderly citizens and act as watchdogs for its use.

The major share of the health care of the elderly in nursing homes is carried out by nurses. The medical profession, in general, does not educate their practitioners for geriatric care (U.S. Congress, 1972), and the level of the profession's interest in this segment of society, unless the patient is in an acute-care facility, seems negligible. Some medical schools are revising their curriculum to include gerontology, but the results will not be appreciated for some time.

The nursing profession has recently expanded required courses in geriatric care, as well as providing nurse-practitioner courses and specialty education. The result is as Roland Yarling (1977) has stated:

> The two professions have evolved in such a way that it is now possible to say, without too much distortion, that, in general, physicians specialize in diseases and nurses specialize in patients. Most frequently, when nothing more can be done about a disease, a great deal more can be done for the patient. And characteristically it is the nurse who does it.

The largest responsibility for geriatric care has been thrust upon the nursing profession. It has accepted the responsibility although it has very little authority for planning, financing, or evaluating the results. However, the profession of nursing is beginning to recognize its power, and the public must be made aware that better care would be possible if more decision-making power were allotted to nursing.

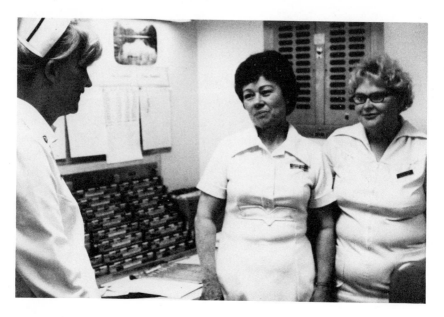

Photographer: Doris Wilson, RN
Models: Dorothy Bison, Lavaughn Kohl, Ava Miles

The licensed practical nurse gives direction and guidance to nursing assistants.

Because geriatric care is primarily nursing care, and because all levels of nursing personnel are required, the practical nurse, even though under the supervision of a registered nurse, has more opportunity for independence and creativity than in any other aspect of nursing at this time.

In many instances the Licensed Practical Nurse is the charge nurse on a unit and is responsible for the care given by nursing assistants. The variety of nursing measures she is required to perform is usually greater than that found in an acute-care facility, where there is more specialization and role definement.

In 1975, 17.3 percent of the practicing LPN/LVNs were employed in nursing homes, second in number only to those employed in hospitals (Kreps, 1978). Hopefully, at some time in your career as a Licensed Practical Nurse, you will decide to seek employment in an institution for the care of the elderly adult.

Nursing in the long-term care facility is especially recommended for those persons who would like to work more independently, feel they have leadership potential, and have a firm grasp of nursing principles and techniques. The more relaxed pace of the nursing home, compared with the acute-care area, is also attractive to many persons.

In the nursing education of today, the common complaint of employers, instructors, and students is the lack of practical experience prior to completion of their nursing courses. It seems that the wisest course for the new graduate is to seek her first position in a hospital. Here she will, under the guidance and assistance of the in-service department and registered nurses, have an opportunity to practice a wide variety of nursing skills and techniques and relate to patients and peers as a Licensed Practical Nurse rather than as a student. A period of transition from the student role is accepted by the nursing service in a hospital, but it may not be provided for in a long-term facility, where responsibility is too great and supervision too limited for a new graduate to cope with. An absence of adequate role models may also deprive the new graduate of favorable learning experiences.

As a Licensed Practical Nurse (hopefully with at least two years' experience) seeking employment in a long-term care facility, what are some of the questions you should have in mind for an employment interview? This interview should never be a one-sided conversation. As a prospective employee, you should be prepared to fulfill your position as an LPN to the best of your ability, in accordance with your education and experience. You must fill out applications and submit recommendations and proof of current licensure. In turn, the facility should be prepared to demonstrate to you what type of operation they conduct. Your professional responsibility is great, and your reputation and retention of your license is your livelihood. If the facility will jeopardize any of these, you do not want to be employed there.

From your nursing classes you will learn the responsibilities of the Licensed Practical Nurse as described in your state's statutes, which are the responsibility of the State Board of Nursing to enforce. While there are not many differences from state to state, there are some, and it is the duty of the licensee to be aware of these rules and regulations.

With the knowledge of her state's rules, the nurse, in her interview with the administrator and/or director of patient care, should ask to read over the job description for the position for which she is applying. Nothing in the job description should be contrary to the state's rules and regulations for practice of nursing by the Licensed Practical Nurse. It should also contain no duties or functions that are contrary to the principles of nursing that she has been taught.

The philosophy of the institution is a statement describing the goal of care toward which they strive and their general beliefs about the people they serve. Nursing service should also have a written philosophy, which is a statement of beliefs about nursing. A set of objectives or goals that describe how the philosophy will be carried out is also helpful in assisting you to understand what kind of care is being given, and what is supposed to be given. Written policies and procedures give directions about how specific situations are to be handled and how nursing techniques are to be carried out (Weber, 1972).

If the job description, philosophy, policy, and procedures are not available for your examination, it will be an indication of poor management, which will probably be reflected in other areas of care.

Personnel policies should describe such items as provision for sick leave, vacation, insurance benefits, holidays, normal shift hours, provision for injury on the job, uniform requirements, and other job-related information. It should also describe the type and amount of in-service education available to the employee through the institution, which is very important for the continued growth of the individual. If your state has a mandatory number of hours of education for licensure, what provision for released time will be made for you to acquire the necessary hours of credit?

Naturally, one of the most important factors is what wage will be paid. The fair wage should be closely correlated with that of a comparable position in an acute-care facility. If you have recently moved, and are unaware of wage scales in the new area, call a nearby hospital, state employment office, or the office of the State Board of Nursing. The applicant should have clear answers to what her monthly salary will be, whether there is a probationary period, when and on what basis are salary increases given, and when and by whom she will be evaluated.

The practical nurse applicant should be prepared to show her current license, list her experience, and have the names and addresses of her sources of recommendations available. She does not need to disclose her religion, marital status, nor age if she does not wish to.

The nurse should not expect, upon seeking a new position, to dictate which shift she will work. In most areas, the supply of both registered and practical nurses is large enough for the facility to choose their prospective employees. The nurse must either meet the facility's need or seek employment elsewhere.

CARE FACILITIES FOR THE ELDERLY ADULT

When the average citizen thinks of the care of the elderly, in most instances he thinks of the nursing home. Only 25 percent of the elderly in the United States are institutionalized; the remainder are either wholly independent or are receiving assistance in programs that allow a larger degree of independence than does the usual long-term care facility. This does not mean that all elderly persons have their needs for health care, housing, food, and other necessities met. These needs have not yet been clearly defined, nor has the percentage of the population in need been identified. They remain the hidden part of a gigantic iceberg.

One of the reasons we do not know exactly how many people need care in institutions is that only the persons actually in residence at any one time are counted; the numbers on waiting lists are not included. Others may be receiving inadequate care or no care at all. It has been estimated that at least twice the number of the elderly now in nursing homes are cared for at home, although they are severely disabled and may require intensive nursing care.

Many elderly Americans continue to maintain a household regardless of their age. The ability to remain independent depends upon many factors; the most common is the mental and physical health of the couple or individual. In some instances, economics or the inability to care for themselves force the couple or individual to sell their home. If there is no low-cost housing available, the elderly couple may move in with their children; which may mean that they are forced to relocate away from friends and all that is familiar to them. This change in arrangements places additional strain on the younger family, who may have difficulties in coping with this adjustment.

Statistics indicate that more than one million elderly persons are cared for in long-term facilities. It is believed that between 14 and 25 percent are placed in facilities that are above the level of their need for care. In almost every instance, the persons who are able to continue to live in their own familiar dwellings are happier and retain more social contacts than those who must be cared for in impersonal surroundings. Life still has a purpose when routine care of the home, gardening, cooking, and laundry must be done. All of these tasks require movement and physical stimulation. They keep one interested and alert. To have all the chores of daily living taken care of, in a manner not prescribed by one's desires, must lead to mental and physical stultification.

Frequently the death of a spouse results in the survivor being forced to seek care elsewhere. This is more common if the survivor is a man; although there are exceptions, female survivors seem to fare better than the male because cooking and housetending chores are more familiar to the female. These skills, as well as the psychological rewards they offer, seem beneficial to the successful coper. In most instances, if a variety of community services are available to assist the elderly, they can stay in their homes for longer periods of time.

Care in the Home

Some elderly couples (or singles) can continue to stay in their homes if they can get assistance for some portion of their daily needs. It may be for such things as heavy cleaning, laundry, or shopping. It might also be for more personal problems. Perhaps partial paralysis, amputations, excessive weight, or lack of strength makes bathing, shampooing or nail care difficult or impossible for elderly adults. They may also have arthritis, cardiac problems, or a terminal illness. Homemaker's services, which are usually contracted for by the hour, are ideal to meet these demands for part-time assistance.

Homemaker- home-health aids work for a community agency and do those tasks that are assigned by a health professional who has assessed the need for services and implements and coordinates the care. In most instances, such programs offer both homemaker and health care services, but they may be offered separately. Health-care services are usually for those requiring professional nursing care, but nursing assistants may also be employed for simple, routine care as Home Health Aides under the direction of a professional. Health-care services enable patients to return home more rapidly after hospitalization and prevent the need for interim care in nursing homes.

The need for homemaker services is greater than the number of certified agencies. The National Council of Homemaker—Home Health Aides Services, Inc. estimates a need for 300,000 aides or one for every 1,000 Americans under 65 years and one for every 100 of those over 65 years. In 1976, there was one homemaker for every 5,000 persons in the country. This care greatly reduces the amount of money that would need to be spent if the elderly adult were housed in a long-term care facility.

Day-care Centers

Day care for the elderly provides a service that enables the participant to stay in his own home or his alternate home (usually a relative's) and will improve the quality of both his and his family's lives and prevent him from having to enter a long-term facility until all other alternatives for care have been exhausted.

Not all persons are eligible for admission to day-care programs. Some of the common criteria are: (1) the applicant must not be harmful to himself or others; (2) he must have a home to return to at night; (3) he must be free from contagious disease; and (4) he must be continent, or be able to attend to his own needs.

The programs should be available at least five days per week, with hours that attempt to correlate with the working hours of the employed family. Participants can choose regular attendance, part-time attendance, or use the day-care center for emergency drop-in only.

The greatest advantage of day-care centers is that by providing a variety of stimulating activities and the opportunity to interact with numerous other persons in a new environment, mental deterioration can be prevented or reversed to some degree. Ideally, the program will also provide health surveillance, health instructions, and suitable activities that will retard physical deterioration. The program offered will depend on the number and variety of staff employed. These programs emphasize retraining and expanding the elderly person's independence. The attitude seems more positive than that of institutional care, as it builds on abilities rather than dwelling on disabilities. Day-care programs are not only beneficial for the elderly, they are much less expensive than care in nursing homes. This reduction in the cost of care affects everyone, because our tax dollars are the source of care for many elderly persons, and we want the best methods used to assure the care and safety of the elderly.

Institutional Care

Nursing homes that are certified for Medicare–Medicaid patients are prepared to give two levels of care: skilled care—in which patients receive professional nursing care 24 hours per day—and intermediate care—which is much less intense than the care of the skilled facility, and where registered nurses may not be present for all shifts. Patients are admitted to these facilities by order of a physician, who decides which level of care is needed by the patient. Most admissions are made following hospitalization, but some are made directly as a result of the physician's private practice, clinic, outpatient department, or other health-care organization.

Most states have other designations for facilities that provide room and board in a protective atmosphere: they may be called congregate-care facilities, domiciliary-care, residential-care, or the like.

The "skilled" nursing home has the highest requirements by law and is prepared to offer the most complex, comprehensive nursing and other types of health care and rehabilitation. Generally speaking, the following types of service are included in nursing-home care.

Primary Service

Primary services are those that are offered by all long-term care facilities. They include care and/or assistance with all activities of daily living (ADL). Food, bathing, clean linen, diet, and exercise are examples of these basic services.

Medical Service

All facilities require that a patient have a designated physician and that he does a complete history and physical examination of the patient, which becomes part of his or her permanent record.

Medications are given by nursing personnel, or the patient takes his own, under supervision, depending upon the level of care he requires.

Rehabilitative services are varied. They may be as simple as exercise classes, range of motion, or they may involve language therapists and physical therapists. The goals may be varied, such as reduction of malfunction, improvement of or maintenance of function.

Psychosocial and social needs of the patients are met by such departments as occupational or recreational therapy, social services, religious services, and a variety of diversional activities.

Operation of the Facility

A long-term nursing facility is a business. The buildings, furnishings, and equipment require large expenditures. Maintenance and labor costs demand additional monies.

Facilities are of three basic types: proprietary, nonprofit, and public. Proprietary homes are privately owned and are expected to return a profit on the investment for the owners. Nonprofit organizations are usually owned by churches, communities, fraternal organizations, and others. Their goal is service, and they are not intended to make a profit. They must, however, return enough earnings to cover the costs of expenditures. If they are unable to do this, they must be supported by some means, such as endowments, gifts, or payment of the deficit by some group. Public facilities are those sponsored by government entities such as counties, large cities, and the federal government. Their goal is service to the specific group of people they serve, and they are financed by public tax monies.

Most proprietary and nonprofit nursing homes have a board of directors composed of members of the community in which they exist. Public nursing homes usually have boards comprised of persons in the governmental bodies that operate the facilities.

The board of directors should reflect the normal mix of the population of the community. The board should include nonprofessionals as well as professional people, and it should have both male and female representation. If the home is operated by religious or fraternal orders, lay persons who have no connection with the operating group should be included. Decisions reached by a variety of persons are usually less biased in any one direction than decisions made by a more homogeneous group.

Factors that Help Insure Good Care

The board of directors, as mentioned previously, can be instrumental in defining realistic, patient-centered goals and attempting to meet community needs. The board of directors and the administrator are legally liable for the care and safety of the patients in the facility.

Many citizens become irate about the care given in nursing homes. As in all other phases of life, there are excellent facilities, and there are average and poor facilities. The best way to insure good care is for consumers of the service (this includes all of us as potential patients) and public groups to keep informed of the level of care, and demand that the homes become accountable for their services. We have this right and responsibility because we (the taxpayers) support these businesses, whether they are proprietary, nonprofit, or public.

The more visitors, students, family, and community volunteers that are present in these facilities, the better will be the care. When institutions operate in isolation, there is a temptation to relax standards, no matter how good the intent. Constant observation demands excellence of care.

Some communities employ an ombudsman for health care, who hears citizens' complaints about health care. The ombudsman visits the facility and the patient or whoever is concerned, and attempts to mediate the problem. In many instances, the issue is one of blocked communication or a misunderstanding.

One ombudsman received a complaint from a relative of an elderly adult that the patients in a certain nursing home were receiving as their source of protein only the game or fish that the administrator, who hunted and fished, provided. Considering the fact that there were 50 patients, the administrator had to be bagging illegal amounts to obtain sufficient quantity to feed the patients. When approached about the complaint, the man was stunned, and stated he occasionally was able to treat a few patients at a time and they enjoyed it. Explanations all around helped solve a situation that hurt a number of people, based upon insufficient knowledge.

Anything that can be done to dispel the isolation and boredom of the residents of an institution helps the people lead a more normal life. The average stay of nursing-home residents is two years, although some are there ten years or more. Few really expect to leave; few have any alternatives available. To adapt successfully to this new home, they must be stimulated by meaningful activities. In some instances, so many activities are available that one wonders how the residents can fit in all the functions in which they are engaged. Having a choice about how one's time is spent is a great morale booster.

Sheltered workshops are present in some homes, where the residents may be stuffing envelopes, addressing them, or packaging small articles for a small wage paid by a local business. Study groups may be formed, and literature, the Bible, or a foreign language may be the focus of the group. Frequent outings such as picnics, ball games, theatre, or the circus may be enjoyed. Some residents are foster grandparents and are literally adopted by a family. Many facilities have monthly dances, weekly bingo, and other activities that are shared with the elderly living in the community. These activities give the residents something to look forward to, and keep social-interaction skills polished as well as promoting some degree of physical activity.

Patient governments or councils—where the residents elect their own officers, who meet regularly with the administration and among themselves—are quite popular. Such a group makes some decisions, listens to complaints of fellow residents, makes and enforces rules, and provides a method of fighting against powerlessness, thereby providing self-esteem.

Nursing homes are often wrongfully blamed for many instances of poor care. The care of the elderly is not only the responsibility of the institution, but of all citizens, who must be informed and sensitive to the problems inherent in the care of the elderly adult.

The Hospice Movement

Hospice is defined as a house of shelter or rest for pilgrims, children, strangers, or the destitute, usually run by religious orders. The hospice is one of the oldest types of institutions for the care of the sick or dying and probably dates to the crusades. Some of the hospices operated by religious orders have endured since those early days.

The hospice movement has been revived recently to give better, more humane care to the terminally ill. These new hospices are not necessarily run by specific religious orders, but are based upon the Christian philosophy of care.

Through the tremendous advances of medical knowledge, we are able to prolong life to a far greater extent than previously thought possible. Potent medication and elaborate machines assist in keeping one alive, and there is a large variety of medications that prevent pain. This combination of machines, drugs, and procedures results in people who are not fully aware of life and whose bodies are invaded by tubes and wires. To many patients and professional health-care givers, such treatment robs the person of human dignity, and the result will still be death. To many, prolonging life, when the situation is terminal, is wasteful of money, health-care hours and facilities, and of the individual's freedom. The entire philosophy of extreme measures seems to dispute the reality of death.

Hospice care accepts death as the normal final cycle of life, and is devoted to the care of the person living out the final phase, rather than just existing. Rather than artificially prolonging life, the patient is kept as comfortable and as active as possible. In a facility that does not deny death, the patient has the peace to grow spiritually and personally during this last experience.

Some of the treatments for malignancies, such as chemotherapy, are continued in a hospice. The medications may cause extreme nausea and vomiting, which results in loss of appetite and strength. Pain is also experienced by many during the terminal phases of their disease. To combat both these problems, medication formulas have been devised that will keep the patient comfortable and free of nausea. In the acute hospital, narcotics, anti-emtics and powerful tranquilizers are given mostly on a PRN (as needed, desired) basis, and if the pain occurs prior to the medication time, one must wait for the designated time to elapse before another dose. Patients are reluctant to ask for medication even when in pain, for fear of addiction or disapproval. When the medications are given frequently, they may reduce the patient to a state of vegetation. He cannot make final plans nor enjoy family visits—he only exists. The hospice formulas are given routinely. The patient is kept free from pain, but is able to move about, think lucidly, and carry on his life as he desires.

Hospices are usually intended for persons with life expectancies of several months. Admissions are very selective because at this time the demand far outreaches the available space.

In some areas, hospice care is given not in an institution, but as a service to terminally ill persons in the home. There may also be a home service connected with an institutional hospice and the person in need may be maintained at home until he needs more constant attention.

It has been found that many persons facing death do not fear the termination of life—they fear the idea of severe, prolonged pain, when they will lose control of their bodies and emotions. Thus, the assurance of freedom from pain and care by people who will allow them to talk about death and their fears is most comforting. The assurance that they will not lose control and will be "themselves" makes the hospice very desirable in contrast to dying in an acute care hospital.

The care given in hospices is primarily nursing care, although medical care is available. Additional medical measures are not attempted unless the patient's condition improves and further treatment seems to be indicated. The philosophy is that unnecessary vigorous treatment that removes the patient from family, reality, and human contact is poor service to the terminally ill.

At present, few hospices exist, although public knowledge about them creates a need. The cost of this type of care is far lower than that of an acute hospital or a long stay in a nursing home. It is certainly more fitted to the needs of many dying persons and is not exclusively for the elderly patient.

The Elderly Isolate

In our society, there is a growing number of elderly adults who would never fit the stereotyped picture of the "grandparent." As in the younger segment of society, there are persons who have never fitted into the main social stream of their community. Many are persons who have had transient jobs, or who have been petty criminals, alcoholics, or prostitutes, or who have never married or had close relatives. Many people who have no close family ties are suspicious of society and its representatives. Most prize their independence highly and will not seek out the various helping programs available, or they may be completely ignorant of them. Many live in highly populated, deteriorated city areas in cheap hotels or walk-up flats. While most persons value independence, these persons isolate themselves for protection and are willing to suffer and die alone for its sake.

Elderly persons face a very real danger from society's abuse, such as mugging, beatings, and other violent crimes. Their awareness of these dangers adds to their lack of trust and their fear of close association with anyone, regardless of the intent of the other persons.

The problems of those in single-room occupancies (SROs) are unknown to most health workers and local authorities. It has been a widely accepted truism that the elderly will accept institutionalization if it is the only method by which they can receive medical and nursing care. Stevens, in her study, indicates that some will refuse assistance rather than jeopardize their independence (Stevens, 1976).

REVIEW QUESTIONS

1. List at least two current problems of the elderly adult and some of the reasons for the occurrence of these problems.

2. Mrs. Nellie Jones, a 72-year-old widow, has poor vision. She recently broke her right arm and is about to be discharged from the hospital. What type of care would you recommend for her and why?

3. List at least three concerns other than salary that the practical nurse should have when applying for a position in a long-term care facility.

4. List some instances when institutionalization is the best approach for care of the elderly adult.

BIBLIOGRAPHY

Anderson, O. W. "Reflections on the Sick Aged and Helping System." *Journal of Gerontological Nursing* 3 (1977): 14–20.

Campbell, M. E. "Study of the Attitudes of Nursing Personnel toward the Geriatric Patient." *Nursing Research* 20 (1971): 147–151.

Dunlap, Burton D. "Need for and Utilization of Long-Term Care among Elderly Americans." *Journal of Chronological Disease* 29 (February 1976): 75–87.

Gollesman, Leonard E., and Norman C. Bauestom. "Why Nursing Homes Do What They Do." *The Gerontologist* 14 (December 1974): 501–506.

Halleck, Seymour. "Why They'd Rather Do Their Own Thing." *Think* 34 (September/October, 1968): 3–7.

Hayter, Jean. "Positive Aspects of Aging." *Journal of Gerontological Nursing* 2 (January/February 1976): 19–23.

Kalish, Richard A. *Late Adulthood: Perspectives on Human Development.* Monterey, Calif.: Brooks/Cole Publishing Co., 1975.

Kleh, Jack. "When to Institutionalize the Elderly." *Hospital Practice* 12 (February 1977): 121–125.

Kreps, Karen. "Practical Nursing—Past, Present and Future." *Nursing Care* 2 (June 1978): 13–22.

Lawton, M. Powell. "Institutions and Alternatives for Older People." *Health and Social Work.* 3 (May 1978): 109–134.

Lorenzee, E. J. et al. "The Day Hospital: An Alternative to Institutional Care." *Journal of the American Geriatrics Society* 22 (July 1974): 316–320.

Miller, Patricia. "RX for the Aging Person: Attitudes." *Journal of Gerontological Nursing* 2 (March/April 1976): 22–26.

Nash, Bernard E. "New Dimensions in the Care of the Aging." *Hospital Progress* 12 (December 1970): 69–72.

Novick, Louis J. "Day Care Meets Geriatric Needs." *Hospitals* 47 (November 1973): 47–50.

O'Brien, Carole Lium. "Exploring Geriatric Day Care: An Alternative to Institutionalization?" *Journal of Gerontological Nursing* 3 (September/October 1977): 26–28.

Pierotte, Doris L. "Day Health Care for the Elderly." *Nursing Outlook* 25 (August 1977): 519–523.

Roby, Frederick B. "Aging and Action." *Western Care* 12 (August, 1970): pp. 14–23.

Standevin, Muriel V. "Social Sensitivity in Health Care." *Nursing Outlook* 25 (October 1977): 640-643.

Stevens, Joyce. *Loners, Losers, and Lovers, Elderly Tenants in a Slum Hotel.* Seattle: University of Washington Press, 1976.

Stoddard, Sandol. *The Hospice Movement.* Briarcliff Manor, N.Y.: Stein and Day, 1978.

U.S. Department of Health, Education and Welfare: Health Services and Mental Health Administration: Washington, D.C.: Government Printing Office. *Biological, Psychological and Social Aspects of Aging,* 1972.

U.S. Congress, Senate, Subcommittee on Long Term Care. *Nursing Home Care in the U.S.: Failure of Public Policy.* Introductory Report. Washington, D.C.: U.S. Printing Office, 1974.

Weber, Helen I. "Written Policies—Insurance for Quality Control." *Nursing Home* 2 (February 1972): 20–22.

Yarling, Roland R. "The Sick Aged, the Nursing Profession, and the Larger Society." *Journal of Gerontological Nursing* 3 (March/April 1977): 42–51.

chapter 2

The Aging Process

OBJECTIVES

After studying this unit, the student will be able to:

1. Describe the normal body changes of the elderly adult.

2. List three factors that are usually true of long-lived persons.

3. Answer some questions the elderly might have about sexual activity.

4. Formulate a standard card plan that could be individualized for a blind person and for one with impaired hearing.

5. List several points that refute the myth that intellect naturally decreases with age.

CHARACTERISTICS OF LONG-LIVED PEOPLE

Why do some people live longer than others? No theory can answer this question accurately for every elderly person. Perhaps more than with any other age group, we tend to lump all "old people" into one anonymous group. But "old people," categorized so from 55 years on, are individuals, each with his own unique physical and personality differences. No one theory can explain all of the various factors that are responsible for aging in the vast variety of elderly people in our population.

The number of older people in the United States has grown approximately 18 percent since 1900; the general population, 13 percent, according to Census Bureau estimates. The greatest growth of the elderly population has been in those states that enjoy a mild, sunny climate. Most older Americans are under 75; half are under 73; a third are under 70. Almost 1.3 million are 85 or over (Spencer, Dorr, 1975, p. 141).

In every country we read of the birthdays of century-old citizens, but there are areas of the world where there are larger than average numbers of persons living to 100 or more years: Ecuador, Kashmir, and some Russian provinces are among the best known. In interviews and studies of these persons, as well as in other investigations, some of the following characteristics of these centarians have been noted.

In most societies, females were found to live from three to seven years longer than males. This appears to be a sex-linked cause. How long this advantage will last, as women smoke more, perhaps drink more, and assume positions of greater responsibility with increased tensions, is a subject of current interest.

The centarians led contented lives and were not worriers. In the societies investigated, no mandatory retirement age was recognized. Regardless of age, the elderly led very active lives. The majority remained free from illness most of their lives and did not have access to modern medical care. Most of them seemed to have normal sex lives and happy or at least comfortable marriages. Interest in sex was maintained throughout life. Dietary investigation showed that their diets were far below the average American caloric intake and contained little animal fat. Most of the persons were slender and strong.

In all of the societies reported on, elderly people were regarded as valued members of society and had a high status in their communities. Most reported that their parents had also lived to an advanced old age. The people were accustomed to doing heavy labor and continued to be very active in their later years. Some observers of the

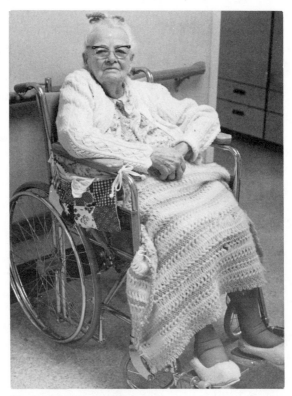

Photographer: Doris Wilson, RN
Model: Alice E. Hallmark

Ninety-nine and one-half years need not diminish one's interest in life.

long-lived Caucasians believe that the studies indicate that hereditary factors protect the person against certain diseases and do not specifically prolong life.

These findings are the result of interviews and observations. Pure scientific research, backed by experimentation, has also increased greatly in the last 20 years. The results indicate that many factors must be considered in the complex phenomena of aging. There is no one simple cause, and there is little agreement among the experts on the causes.

The individual's chronological age is a poor indication of his physiological age. Some of the supposed indicators of old age, such as arteriosclerosis, can be found in twenty-year-olds. One finding is agreed upon by the majority of scientists—that having a background of long-lived ancestors greatly increases one's chances of living to an old age.

Another widely accepted concept of aging is based upon risks to old age. These include air-pollution, obesity, excess use of alcohol and tobacco, and lack of regular exercise. These risks are centuries old, but increase with increased standards of living.

In attempting to list the characteristics of long-lived persons, we find that they are of tremendous variety, just as are those characteristics that we attribute to teenagers, new mothers, or any other segment of society.

PHYSICAL AND FUNCTIONAL CHANGES OF AGING

Elderly people often report, in relating their lives, that "all of a sudden I was old." Children often remark of their parent, "He aged overnight." While the realization that one has aged may seem to occur almost instantaneously, the aging process has been going on since birth, but proceeds at vastly different rates in each person. This is a normal cycle of life; the person ages gradually according to a somewhat prerecorded individual timetable. Some factors of life speed the clock; others slow it. There is no single cause for aging. A combination of several factors will cause the final result—death.

Not all body cells age at the same rate in the same individual. As some cells die, they are not all replaced, particularly in the heart and brain; others, such as skin, mucous membrane, and blood are regularly replaced. In time of stress to the body, the elderly person has less reserve for crisis than does the younger person. These changes may be described as a change in the body's ability to maintain homeostasis, the ability to restore equilibrium or balance to the complex system of the body. The physical changes that we can readily observe are the ones we most frequently associate with old age.

Skin

Elderly persons' skin becomes inelastic and wrinkled as the underlying fatty deposits are lost, and it also becomes thinner and more prone to abrasions and bruises as the underlying vessels also become more fragile. Pigmentary discolorations, sometimes called "liver spots," occur, particularly on the face, neck and hands. These may cause great distress, particularly in women, who see them as very visible signs to the world that they are growing old. Sweating is decreased as sweat glands become more inactive.

Visual Acuity

The reduction of visual acuity is as individual as other changes that occur with age. The change that occurred in middle age, farsightedness, tends to cease its advance. Depth and color discrimination become less acute. Night lights are poorly tolerated, and night driving is difficult or impossible. Cataracts and glaucoma may further the difficulties of the elderly person's vision.

Some elderly adults stop reading or watching television, which restricts their enjoyment of life, with the mistaken idea that they are preserving their failing vision.

Behavioral problems such as irritability or reclusive, "senile behavior" may be caused by loss of visual acuity. In many instances, failure to see clearly is not reported to anyone. The individual feels it is just "part of growing old." With vision corrected, which will aid mobility and independence, behavior may also change, as abilities discarded can once again be pursued. Poor vision, which is so common in the elderly, also goes unnoticed in many instances by nursing personnel because the patient has adapted so well to the absence of acute vision. Some patients who are totally blind require cataract extraction, which may have been overlooked in their care.

Some persons are nursing-home residents for years without having an eye examination. Although a nursing home resident may find it difficult to get to an optometrist (OD) or opthalmologist (MD), the major consideration would seem to be cost: medicare does not finance routine exams or glasses; it provides care only for eye diseases. Medicaid does provide assistance.

Hearing

Some degree of hearing difficulty is reported in 27 percent of persons over 75. Changes in hearing actually begin before 40, when high-pitched tones are no longer heard accurately. Hearing loss in later years occurs for no apparent reason. Persons who have been employed in occupations with a high noise factor suffer hearing loss and deafness most frequently. Boilermakers, railroad engine crews, jackhammer operators and others have hearing-hazardous jobs. Many in such occupations are now required to wear protective ear guards, but government regulations do not cover all the hazards. It may be predicted that present-day musicians who have worked with greatly amplified instruments will be the next generation's hard-of-hearing.

Adequate communication with the patient suffering from hearing impairment is difficult. It may be further complicated by the presence of background noise, which is always with us. The patient's history, daily assessment, and requests may contain erroneous information if the patient has misunderstood the questions put to him.

Problems of communication with persons of varying degrees of deafness can be met in several ways.

1. By raising the voice moderately, by enunciating clearly and more slowly.
2. By written communication.
3. By use of a hearing aid.

Shouting at a patient is not a suitable remedy. The patient can observe your strain, which embarrasses him; it destroys any semblance of privacy, which might be indicated, and it is extremely tiring. It may also be said to be "catching," as the tendency is to shout at everyone.

The use of hearing aids is acceptable to some patients. Others refuse to have testing; 34 percent of the elderly have never had a hearing test. Some refuse to wear an aid because they prefer to deny hearing loss or because they are embarrassed to wear one. The problems of static noise or squeals further the embarrassment of the wearer. When a person has some hearing, an aid can amplify that sound. If nerve deafness is present, amplification will not help, because the sounds being received are garbled.

Most governmental programs do not pay for hearing aids, so many needy persons are denied their assistance. Hearing aids are powered by batteries, which are expensive and must be replaced frequently; patients often become disgusted with the aid when battery-power is at fault. Hearing aids not only amplify speech, they also pick up extraneous noises and amplify them. This proves so upsetting to some, accustomed as they are to quiet, that they either turn off the aid or refuse to wear it. Ear molds or earpieces must fit properly and be positioned correctly or the sounds from earpieces will be amplified in a high-pitched squeal from the microphone.

The nurse can assist the hard-of-hearing patient best if she faces him, allowing the patient to see her face and lips clearly. The voice should be only moderately raised, and the speech should be clearly and slowly enunciated. When communications are imperative, some patients can profit by use of a stethoscope—the nurse speaks into the bell, while the earpieces are in the patient's ears.

One of the gravest side effects of loss of hearing is the exclusion from normal communication. To see people talking, and not hear, makes one feel that they are whispering, and the conclusion is easily reached that the matter concerns oneself. Anger, suspicion, and disengagement may follow. Paranoia develops easily from such incidents, and isolation from life becomes more pronounced, as the person refuses to interact with others.

Voice

The elderly person may notice voice changes, as the voice seems to lose strength and become lower in volume and slower.

Taste

A common comment of the older adult concerning food is, "It just isn't as good as it once was." While this may be true of differences in preparation and freshness, it is also true that the sense of smell deteriorates, which has much to do with our enjoyment of food. The number of taste buds also diminishes, and they are not replaced, so taste is less acute and may account for some of the changes noticed by the individual.

Ambulation

If one observes people walking along the street without observing their faces, it is possible to identify the elderly solely by their gait and stride. The pace of the older person is slower and may become an uneven, shuffling gait. Endurance is reduced, and we see sidewalk benches or shopping-mall rest areas used frequently by older persons. The muscle fibers have been reduced and are less elastic. Formerly erect posture may change to an unattractive stoop due to changes in the spine, where bones are more porous, and arthritic changes occur where the intervertebral disks no longer adequately cushion the vertebrae. In women, a hump, called the "dowager's hump or buffalo hump." may appear between the shoulders. Joints stiffen due to changes in the lining of the joint cavity, and kneeling, bending, and elbow movement become slow and painful or nearly impossible. These skeletal changes are particularly serious, as any problem that reduces activity accelerates other changes.

Metabolism

The body's ability to utilize food efficiently is decreased with advancing years. People tend to retain their habitual diet, and unless body activity is maintained at its earlier level, the excess food consumed is stored as fat, which may further impede activity. Additional weight puts strain on the deteriorating joints, and causes additional pain and stiffness. The increased weight may decrease coordination and be a factor in increased falls, particularly in the female, although this may also be attributed to deterioration of the vestibular senses.

Deposition of fat around the heart interferes with its normal function, and the blood pressure rises. Obesity affects the circulatory system and the kidneys. The metabolism of sugar is impeded, and the resulting diabetes, unless quickly and consistently controlled, results in further physiological complications, deterioration, and reduction of life span.

Oral Changes

Tooth and gum changes occur and there are numerous problems. While some elderly persons retain their teeth until very late in life or until death, more than 50 percent of the people over 65 years are edentulous.

Sexual Activity

One of the myths about the elderly adult is that sexual expression is not necessary past a given age. This magic age probably varies according to the interpreter. If it is your parent in question, the age of ceasing sexual activity may be placed as early as forty. Certainly society in general believes it to be the late middle years or slightly later.

If society observes that there is evidence of sexual activity in the elderly person, it may be viewed with disgust, outrage, or amusement. These attitudes are repeated endlessly in bad jokes, cartoons, and other media presentations. Marriage of very elderly persons is newsworthy. Regardless of the extent to which our mores tolerate sexual freedom, these freedoms are reserved for the younger age group and are not tolerated in the elderly. Not only are the young people of our society misinformed about sex in the later years, the elderly are also ignorant of the sexual potentiality. If the older person has sexual needs, he must stifle them or run the risk of societal condemnation. Disregarding these needs may lead to feelings of frustration, guilt, and anger.

While research on all aspects of sexuality has been accelerated in the past decade, relatively little research has been done with the aged. What has been discovered is that there is no physiological reason that satisfying sexual activity cannot continue throughout life.

Masters and Johnson and Kinsey report that after age 18, the male's sexual peak begins to decline. Women's peak years occur in the 30s and 40s, but their decline is slower than the rate for males.

Sex practices of the elderly generally follow the patterns of earlier life. Those who were very active tend to remain so in later life. Those with weaker sexual urges cease functioning. Many males, who mistakenly believed that "saving" their sexual potency would enable it to last longer in life, may have a difficult or impossible task when they wish to become active again.

The female, although she undergoes some body changes, such as reduction of vaginal lubrication and a tendency to irritation of the thinner vaginal tissue, nevertheless is capable of orgasm regardless of age. Sexual activity can be restarted at any time, although some initial discomfort may occur until the activity again becomes more frequent.

The male, as stated, does have changes in his sexual ability, but it is more or less in relationship to other changes, such as strength and endurance, and is part of normal aging. Because of myths about sexual decline in later years, he may have fears that seem to be commonly identified by males, such as (1) not having adequate erections; (2) premature ejaculation; (3) inability to retain erection; and (4) inability to satisfy the sex partner.

If the elderly male can be assured that intercourse is possible throughout life, although its character may not be comparable to his performance at age 20 or 30, this period of time, when his mate is free of worry about childbearing, can be the most satisfying and lead to the closest relationship of their life. The power of self-fulfilling prophecies must be recognized. If the wife insists that her mate is too old for sex or he becomes convinced that this part of his life is over, the fallacies may indeed become a certainty.

The Brain

The brain does not undergo major changes with aging. It continues to function well if there is no disease and if it continues to receive adequate oxygen and nutrition through normal circulation. Certain chemicals, including alcohol and drugs, can damage the brain.

Circulation to the brain is greatly affected by cerebral vascular accidents (stroke), which may occur suddenly. Atherosclerosis is caused by fatty deposits in the vessels with elastic media, that is, the coronary arteries, the aorta and main branches, and the larger arteries of the brain. These deposits cause reduction in the lumen of the vessels; the walls of the vessel become rough so that thrombosis (clots) may form and the walls become so thin that aneurysms (out-pouching) or rupture of the artery may occur.

When loss of brain function occurs from atherosclerosis, some of the specialized functions of the cerebrum are changed. Memory, judgment, and personality may change. These alterations may occur so gradually they may be undetectable for some time. Eventually, memory lapses, sudden dozing off, irritability, and many verbal repetitions of statements occur.

If atherosclerotic changes in the brain are combined with hypertension, the rupture of a blood vessel is more likely. Cerebrovascular accidents (CVAs) may be fatal, or they may be so slight as to be unnoticed. Cerebrovascular accidents do not suddenly affect intellect, but they may affect the patient's ability to speak and to move. Speech is controlled by "handedness," and will be affected by the side of the brain on which the vascular damage occurs. If the person is ambidextrous, he has some speech area on both sides of the brain and will not lose all speech.

The effects of a CVA can be reversed to a variety of degrees, depending upon the initial severity and the determination of the patient as well as the caliber of help he receives. Never count a patient out because of a CVA, and do not assume there is a lack of intelligence if the patient cannot speak. Rehabilitation requires patience, persistence, and a positive attitude. Success may not be accomplished to the degree one wishes, but any functional recovery will help the patient to lead a more normal life with courage to continue the therapy required.

There are some diseases that are more prevalent in the later years where cell loss and brain atrophy occur. Some appear early, in the late forties or fifties, others occur late, and are labeled "senility," but really are diseases. Dementia will be discussed more fully in Chapter 3.

The Heart

Cardiovascular disorders are the leading cause of death in the United States. Many elderly persons have cardiac diseases, but many also have abnormal cardiorespiratory functions, which result from the normal aging process.

As the body ages, the blood vessels lose their elasticity, become hardened, lengthen, and become more tortuous. This is a normal change, and the rate and severity varies with the individual. As the lumen of the vessel decreases, both the systolic and diastolic blood pressure rises. As the patient reduces his normal activities, his metabolic rate also decreases, and with arteriosclerosis and perhaps atherosclerosis also present, the muscles of the heart receive less blood supply. This results in a drop in cardiac output, which means that the extremities also receive less blood.

When the person is seated, the lower extremities may become mottled or cyanotic and the feet will be cold. Pedal pulses may be weak. Extreme care must be used so that no clothing restricts circulation and the patient is dressed warmly but lightly. Bed socks may be used, but heat, in the form of hot-water bottles or heating pads, should not be applied, as the patient may be severely burned due to loss of sensitivity to temperature change.

With reduced cardiac output, the patient will fatigue quickly. He must be cautioned concerning activities that put sudden stress on the heart. Sudden demands on the heart may result in cardiac insufficiency. Nursing measures should be planned for short intervals of activity to prevent fatigue.

Reduced cardiac efficiency may result in decrease of blood supply to the brain, which may result in dizziness, confusion, or syncope (fainting).

Elderly persons should be cautioned not to rise suddenly from a recumbent position; they should be taught simple isometric exercises for their feet and ankles before rising first to a seated position and then upright. If they are standing, the exercises can also be done periodically and should be interspersed with periods of being seated. Simple precautions can prevent dangerous falls for the older adult.

Respiratory Changes

The decreased cardiac output also results in a decreased oxygen exchange to all the cells. The lungs fail to work as efficiently, as the bony rib cage becomes less elastic, reducing expansion. Skeletal changes, which cause the posture to change from upright to stooping, further decrease the chest capacity.

Changes in the muscles of respiration also make optimum respiration impossible. The ability to cough effectively is impaired, although increased morning cough is common. The lungs retain some mucus, and respiratory function is lost, while the possibility of infection is increased. Exercise, clean atmosphere, and no smoking can improve lung function. Unfortunately, many older adults have respiratory diseases in addition to the normal changes brought on by increased age.

PERSONAL ADJUSTMENTS TO AGING

Adjustment to the changes and limitations of aging will doubtless follow the manner in which the necessary adjustments of preceding years of life were managed. The beginning of adjustment does not take place at age 60, 65, or 70, but is a subtle adaptation over several decades.

The loss of muscular strength, agility, and speed of movement may be more upsetting to others than it is to the elderly person, as

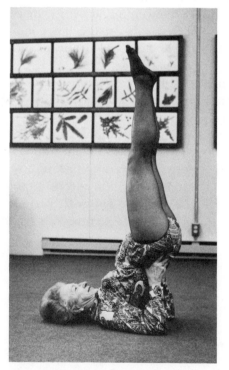

Photographer: Doris Wilson, RN
Model: Helen Ferguson

Sixty-five years do not hinder this woman's physical fitness routine.

he no longer has the same need for these functions as he had at age 30 or 40. He no longer needs to meet society's demand for specific output of energy. Society, however, seems to gauge "successful" aging as that appearance, activity level, and philosophy that most nearly imitates middle age.

Successful adaptation may necessitate the acceptance and acknowledgement that some assistance may be necessary in order to function with the changes that have taken place in one's body. Assistance may be required first for heavy household chores, and later for personal needs. This type of help was necessary during the first cycle of life and should be regarded as normal during the last cycle, differing in time placement and degree for each individual. The difference that should also be appreciated by all is the need for the person in the last cycle of life to retain his independence and to make his own decisions. Adaptation to the later years would no doubt be less stressful if each person could terminate activities in his own time frame and initiate others as he desired, dependent only on his safety to self and others, not upon his chronological age.

The theory of disengagement has a basis in the belief that all die and leave society and preparation for this departure takes the form of a gradual release of power and responsibility. Some of our cultural mores and even laws are based upon this premise. We have ideas about 65-year-olds entering college, how long one should be able to drive, how old one should be to remarry, take one's pension, receive social security, and many other facets of life.

The disengagement theory suggests that the elderly cease their interactions with others and become more self-centered. This theory has been revised by some and discarded by others. There is the connotation that this is an unhealthy approach to one's later years. While this may well be true for many, for others it may be ideal. Some lives have been so full of activities of child rearing, with both parents working, perhaps multiple jobs, doing service to their community and church, that they almost literally had no time for self. Gradual withdrawal from some of these activities and people may be an opportunity to enrich one's inner life, to do one's "own thing." It is also an opportunity to choose one's own contacts—not to play the game of those who must be cultivated and entertained.

One of the most important attributes for successful aging is maintenance of personal dignity. To retain this, one must be able to demand respect. Some persons have no problem, regardless of their age, in speaking out in their own defense. Other persons, who perhaps

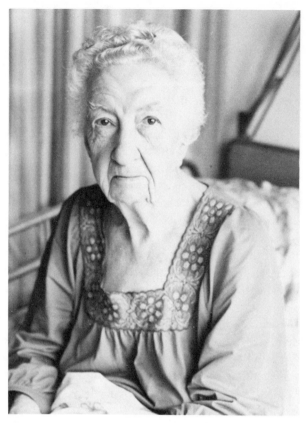

Photographer: Doris Wilson, RN
Model: Irene Saunders

A spirit of "bloody-mindedness" helps one survive.

have never been assertive, get pushed around—both literally and fig-
uratively. Assertive training might be the most valuable tool they
could acquire. Alex Comfort (1976) defines this attribute as "bloody-
mindedness."

> It subsumes feistiness, cussedness and orneriness, with
> overtones of heroic obstinacy in not being put down, in defying
> popes, presidents, priests, professors, pundits and people gener-
> ally when defending your own patch and your own right to be
> yourself. Bloody-mindedness is the chief adaptive character of
> man, . . . and it is the ultimate resource of the senior person.
> (p. 45)

REVIEW QUESTIONS

1. What suggestions would you give to a person who inquires what he can do to survive to advanced years?
2. What methods can you use to facilitate communication with the hard-of-hearing?
3. What answer would you give to a 69-year-old widow who reports sexual inactivity for ten years, who is to be remarried, and asks if sexual intercourse will be possible?
4. Why are elderly adults particularly prone to respiratory infections?
5. Do all elderly patients lose their intellectual abilities as they age?

BIBLIOGRAPHY

"Age Stereotyping and Television." *Committee on Aging*. U.S. House of Representatives, 95th Congress, Washington, D.C., 1977.

Anwar, Masud. "Communication Difficulties with the Elderly Hard-of-Hearing." *Nursing Mirror* 145 (November 3, 1977): 26-29.

Benet, Sula. *How to Live to Be 100*. New York: The Dial Press, 1976.

Chapman, Ruth H. "No Longer at Risk: Sex Among the Elderly." *Family Planning and Perspectives* 8 (September/October, 1976), p. 253.

Comfort, Alex. *A Good Age*. New York: Crown, 1976.

Davies, David. *The Centarians of the Andes*. Garden City, Anchor Press/Doubleday, 1975.

Gardiner, P. A. "Failing Vision in the Elderly." *Nursing Mirror* 145 (November 3, 1977): 29-30.

Griggs, Winona. "Sex and the Elderly." *American Journal of Nursing*. 78 (August 1978): 1352-1354.

Hogstel, Mildred O. "How Do the Elderly View Their World?" *American Journal of Nursing* 78 (August 1978): 1335-1338.

Holm, Carol S. "Deafness: Common Misunderstandings." *American Journal of Nursing* 78 (November 1978): 1910-1912.

Huyck, Margaret Hellie. *Growing Older*. Englewood Cliffs, N.J.: Prentice-Hall, 1974.

Knopf, Olga. Successful Aging—The Facts and Fallacies of Growing Old. New York: The Viking Press, 1975.

McKinley, Hedi, and Belle Drew. "The Nursing Home: Death of Sexual Expression." *Health and Social Work* 2 (August 1977): 180-187.

Moran, Joyce. "Sexuality After Sixty." *Association of Rehabilitative Nurses' Journal* 2 (July/August 1977): 19–21.

Papalia, Diane E., and Sally W. Olds. *Human Development*. New York: McGraw-Hill, 1978.

Schlesinger, Benjamin. "Sexuality and the Senior Citizen." *Canada's Mental Health* 25 (September 1977): 15–16.

Skuka, Burt. "Geriatric Vision Care." *Nursing Care* 9 (April 1976): 26–28.

Smith, Bert Kruger. *Aging in America*. Boston: Beacon Press, 1973.

Spencer, Marian G., and Caroline Dorr, eds. *Understanding Aging*. New York: Appleton-Century-Crofts, 1975.

Spinazzola, Angelo J. "Sexual Patterns in the Process of Aging." *Health Education* 6 (July/August/1975): 11–13.

Twente, Esther. *Never Too Old*. San Francisco: Jossey-Bass Inc., 1970.

Uhler, Diana M. "Common Skin Changes in the Elderly." *American Journal of Nursing* 78 (August 1978): 1342–1344.

chapter 3

Behavior Patterns of the Elderly Adult

OBJECTIVES

After studying this unit, the student will be able to:

1. List several crises experienced by the elderly adult.

2. Define anxiety and describe some of its symptoms and causes.

3. Describe the typical depressed patient and list several common causes for his behavior.

4. Explain when the suicide risk is highest in depressed patients.

5. Describe several methods that will help the potential suicide improve his self-image.

6. Describe the differences between acute and chronic brain syndrome.

7. List several methods of assisting the confused patient to live as normally as possible.

EMOTIONAL AND SOCIAL CRISIS OF THE ELDERLY

Crises may be defined as those times in life when a person cannot solve a problem by using the same methods formerly used to cope with similar problems. The inability to resolve the problem results in anxiety and tension, which, if not relieved, result in emotional and physical deterioration.

Most elderly adults are healthy, both mentally and physically. The crises they face seem to increase with age. As in the beginning of adolescence, the crises of the later years may be grouped into emotional, social, and physical categories. However, no problem consists only of one single factor, and cause cannot be precisely isolated. Some of the more common crises are as follows.

Career Changes

We do not normally think of the elderly as having career changes, but career changes occur frequently when the person has been forced to leave a longtime position due to compulsory retirement or a disability that precludes continuing on a particular job. In most instances, the second career is not as prestigious as the first, and the peer group with whom he has long been associated is lost to him. The need to seek another job is, in itself, frightening, possibly humiliating, when the skills of selling oneself have not been practiced and the person in power may well be years younger and have less experience than the applicant. After normal retirement, many persons seek reemployment because of low fixed incomes or boredom. For persons age 50 and over, a new job will be hard to find. Menial-type jobs may be the only ones available. Pride and self-esteem suffer when these events occur.

45

Death

Fear of death is not peculiar to the aged; its fear is universal in all ages. Many elderly persons experience the death of children, who may themselves be past middle age, but who will always remain "young" to the parents. Friends and public figures die, and upon each occasion, one's own mortality is reemphasized. Regardless of the number of deaths that occur, the ability to cope with this crisis does not improve. It is not uncommon that deaths may occur so rapidly that one does not have time to mourn and recover before another occurs. The death of a longtime spouse is probably as near to being the death of oneself that can occur. The enormous emotional investment one makes in the life of a beloved partner is greater than any other in life.

Health

Adaptation to changes in body functions and in all functions and activity is a long-term process. While the changes may cause severe crises in some persons, others may have difficulty in identifying when they started, so complete is their acceptance. The anticipation of dependency upon others, however, for part or all of one's normal activities and needs, or the sudden occurrence of this catastrophe, is a severe crisis.

Housing

Regardless of the quality of housing, the necessity to change living arrangements after years of occupancy, work, and investment is a severe sacrifice. To leave that comfortable, secure haven to be institutionalized is a sacrifice; it signifies what might be identified as a prematurely published obituary, "this spells the end—my home is gone and I have only numbered days—I will not return home nor to normal life."

Income Reduction

In a society where personal worth is all too often judged by income, the reduction in income as a result of retirement may create a crisis.

Many Americans, regardless of the knowledge of forthcoming retirement, have made no financial plans for the actual cessation of monthly paychecks. Many have no idea how much they will receive from pensions, social security, or other sources. In addition to failure to save during the years of employment, a home may not be paid for and large bills may be outstanding. Retirement may necessitate drastic cutbacks in entertainment, housing, transportation, and clothing.

Regardless of the former level of living, retirement, for all but a few, will necessitate some adjustment of lifestyle at the same time other crises are common. For some, retirement may be a time of actual need and deprivation.

Societal Attitudes

As old age develops, the person who was an active member of his community and family does not feel he is a "different" person, despite the changes in his body and appearance.

What a shock it is when one first understands that an attitudinal change in one's children, neighbors, or colleagues is due to one's age. Did the slow answer to a question about work, a forgotten appointment, white hair, or trouble lifting heavy grocery bags bring about this change? No longer asked to be a committee chairman, no requests for extra work, exclusion from a daughter's bridge game—when did it start? These types of seemingly trivial occurrences may be the beginning of understanding that one is old to others, that one is being differentiated from "regular" society, that one's opinion is of little value to anyone.

An interesting example of attitudes was recently portrayed on a major television game show. Four players (all under 40) were playing a word game where two persons gave clues to the other two to help them recognize the word "retired." The clues given to the players were "over," "jobless," "aged," and "home." The picture of the retired person conjured up was acute. In reality, the retired person could be from 40 to 100 years of age and, regardless of age, an active, vital person.

COMMON TYPES OF BEHAVIOR, OBSERVATIONS AND INTERVENTION

The brief descriptions of crises common to the elderly that, if not resolved, result in anxiety, tension, and eventually physical and mental deterioration are rarely matters that come to the attention of health professionals. Only when the behavior resulting from the crisis is so bizarre and so far outside society's norms that institutional placement is required, is the help of a professional sought.

The behavior exhibited by elderly persons differs little from that of the population as a whole, particularly when facing crisis situations. However, when nurses must care for and assist the elderly in institutions, these behaviors may hinder the care of the patient, or they may be the primary cause of his need for care.

Anxiety and depression are the two most common results of the elderly adult's experiences in a long-term facility. The behaviors that result from unresolved crises vary, and understanding the behavior and assisting the patient to adaptive behavior is crucial in the comprehensive care of the elderly adult.

Anxiety

Anxiety is both chronic and intermittent and is difficult or impossible for the patient to describe. It is an unpleasant feeling of apprehension, helplessness, and uncertainty that makes thinking and acting difficult, if not impossible, depending upon the severity of the feeling. Patients do not usually describe their problem as anxiety, but rather as "not feeling right," "having no energy," or "extreme nervousness." The feeling of undefined dread and mental confusion is extremely uncomfortable. One wants to escape this painful experience but seems unable to proceed in any meaningful fashion. Denial of anxiety is common, and somatic complaints seem more acceptable to the elderly.

In observing the anxious elderly adult, the nurse may make some of the following observations:

- Patients frequently remove themselves from the general interactions of the institution, becoming less verbal and appearing forlorn. This mood may change rapidly: the patient becomes very talkative and seeks out persons never before approached in an effort to form relationships. Restlessness, chain-smoking, and various nervous mannerisms are common.
- Episodes of crying, demanding, and shouting may occur if attention cannot be found in more normal fashion. The anxi-

ous person may be very irritable and take offense easily. Escape into fantasy is frequent: the patient may feel less anxious by escaping from reality.

- Pulse and respiration rates may be accelerated and blood pressure may be elevated. Frequent and urgent urination and, less frequently, diarrhea may occur. With severe anxiety, hyperventilation may occur. Normal patterns of sleeping are disturbed, and tranquilizers or sleeping medications are often requested. Eating habits may also be disturbed, and either loss of appetite or overeating may occur. Direct eye contact may be avoided.

While anxiety may occur at any time, it is frequently found on and following the admission of the elderly adult to the long-term facility.

Millie Tanner had been dead for a year. During that year, Herb Tanner, 78 years old, had tried to do all the things Millie had done to keep their small house so comfortable: cleaning the yard, doing the laundry, cooking, and cleaning the house. At first, neighbors offered to help, and their son, who lived across the county, 60 miles away, visited frequently. His own problems soon decreased the numbers of trips he made.

In the scramble to keep up, doing things only Millie had done, Herb forgot to take his heart pills. Soon the many tasks became too tiring and breathing became difficult. Weeds grew, laundry was forgotten, and meals were eaten only if they were remembered. The world seemed senseless, and Herb felt guilty about the ever-increasing disorder about him. Why had all this been forced on him, when he hadn't even had a chance to grieve for Millie? Slipping on spilled water in the kitchen, Herb broke his arm. A brief hospitalization was necessary and then he was admitted to a nursing home until he was able to move his arm again. Herb was glad to allow others to care for him, but he was also angry because he was dependent. Nurses quickly observed that he was severely anxious. In giving an admitting history, Herb and his son supplied information that gave clues to the causes of the anxiety.

1. Herb had not been able to cope with the sudden death of his wife.

2. His health, due to lack of proper medication and poor nutrition, was a constant concern.

3. He was alone without support from neighbors and family.

4. He felt guilty about his inability to cope with all of the household problems formerly shared with his spouse. He didn't like the tasks he was forced to assume and felt frustrated because he felt he should have been able to do them.

5. He was angry with Millie for deserting him.

6. He had made no plans for the future nor any changes in his routine to help cope with his problems.

7. He definitely was not enjoying life nor did he foresee the future in any favorable terms.

8. He did not want to be in a nursing home and was angry with his son and his doctor, who he felt were to "blame" for his present plight.

Nursing Intervention for Anxiety

If the patient can talk about his anxiety (he may label this as an uncomfortable feeling, "the blahs," or other descriptive variations) and acknowledge its presence, the nurse can affirm that she recognizes the patient's feelings. This affirmation is supportive to the patient and opens the way for further discussions.

If the patient denies anxiety, or is unwilling or unable to express his concerns, regardless of the behavior that made the nurse's observation possible, it should not be discussed further, as anxiety may be greatly increased. Medications appropriate to reducing anxiety should be sought, and after they have become effective, further exploration can proceed.

To obtain information about the causes of anxiety and how the patient coped with the problem in prior occurrences may take a long time or may never be possible. The behavior that is being exhibited as a result of anxiety may be either acceptable or unacceptable.

If the behavior is unacceptable, the nurse must take care that her behavior and that of others does not result in rejection of the anxious person. His behavior should be reported to him as unacceptable and other ways of coping should be explored. Limits can be set.

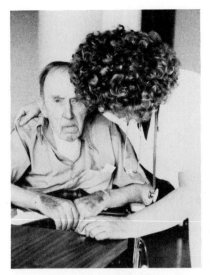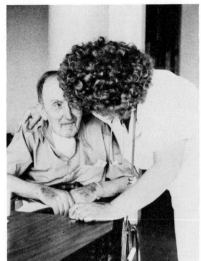

Photographer: Doris Wilson, RN   *Model: William J. McCutcheon*

Before and after a visit and concerned touch by the nurse.

Anxious persons should have other persons near. Ideally, family, friends, and others should be enlisted. Nursing and other personnel can be involved in frequent encounters. Arranging for coffee breaks with other patients or nurses will help him become part of the group. The use of touch beyond that necessary for routine care will help with feelings of self-esteem and soothe the anxious patient. Above all, time set aside for listening to the patient's problems or reminiscences is essential. Taking the problems seriously and assisting the patient to do his own problem solving is beneficial. Assisting with and contributing to reminiscence seems to help the patient gain new perspectives on what has happened to him and to alleviate anxiety.

Depression

Depression is another behavior resulting from unresolved crises. The multiple losses common to the elderly adult may be one of the primary causes of depression. If there is no one available to support the elderly adult and his inner strengths are insufficient to overcome the stress and anxiety of loss, depression may occur.

A common form of depression in the elderly person is a normal reaction following death of a loved one, or loss of anything that has

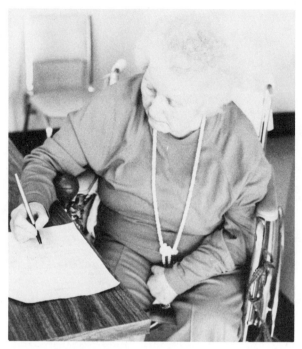

Photographer: Doris Wilson, RN
Model: Minette Walter

A patient signs a photo permission—someone values her contribution.

significant value to one. Failure in an important activity may also cause depression. As time progresses, however, and normal activities are reactivated, depression lifts and other matters preoccupy the mind and the feelings.

Depression may result from an actual or fancied belief that family members or friends no longer care about one's welfare. Elderly adults often experience feelings of guilt and anger, failure and worthlessness, which lead to depression. Whether or not depression will be overcome depends to some degree upon the person's ability in the past to cope with adversities.

Depression, like anxiety, is experienced in degrees. The person may describe that he feels exhausted, vaguely confused, and hopeless. He may worry constantly and relate to himself and others the happenings of long periods of his life in an endeavor to discover what went wrong. In more severe depression, some disorientation may be present as well as poor judgment. The person may be unable to act, although the desire to escape from his depression is strong.

The depressed patient is one who appears sad, whose body seems to droop, who walks slowly, if at all, and whose responses to speech and other stimuli are greatly slowed. Crying is common, and he may clutch at nurses or others in an attempt to relate to others. In more severe depression, the patient may withdraw—seeking privacy— and refuse to talk to or even look directly at others. Dress and personal hygiene may be neglected, and meals may be skipped or intake greatly reduced.

This period is one of reduced self-esteem. One's former abilities seem lost, and the person underachieves. Pessimism and hopelessness are communicated. Speech retardation may occur, and the person is very critical of self.

The symptoms of depression may be wholly emotional, wholly physical, or a combination of both. Any disease process can cause depression, but low blood glucose (hypoglycemia) may also be present. Blood tests may determine if this is the problem. A check also to determine if the depression is always present or becomes more severe at certain hours may indicate that (1) meals are too far apart; (2) meals contain excess carbohydrates and insufficient protein; (3) not enough food is being ingested; or (4) supplementary snacks are necessary.

If nutrition and blood levels are normal, or until the cause can be determined, the depressed patient needs rest and comfort, to overcome fatigue. Rest should not be defined as total bed rest however, as stimulation is needed to maintain sensory function. Judicious use of touch by the nurse and ambulation with assistance, if necessary, will be helpful. Rest and activity should be interspersed.

The nurse should be noncritical during this time and reduce any demands on the patient, as he cannot handle additional stress. Personal hygiene should be stressed, however, and assistance should be provided freely during this time. Any effort should be praised and improvement noted continually. Diversional activities and increased social contacts help the person to feel more positive about himself and the future.

If there are persons available for support, such as family, friends, church members, or members of organizations, these people should be contacted and asked for assistance in helping the patient regain his equilibrium. If these helpers are not available, arrangements for phone calls to relatives may be possible. A senior telephone calling service or members of a senior center may also be involved to help the depressed person to feel that someone cares.

Depression is only abnormal when it is greatly prolonged or when the severity has no realistic cause. A moderate- to severely-depressed person must always be considered a potential suicide and be closely observed and protected to prevent such an act. The greatest danger for suicide is when the person seems to be improving, and depression seems to have lifted. This probably results from the person's decision to end his life. The decision to act seems to relieve tension and reduce worries about the future.

The Suicidal Patient

Suicide was the eighth major cause of death in the United States in 1973. In the population as a whole, the suicide rate was 12 per 100,000. For persons 65 and over, the rate was 23 per 100,000 (Bureau of Census, 1975).

Depression, common in the elderly, is a major cause of suicide in this age group. As previously discussed, depression occurs following crisis, usually a loss or a series of losses. Any occurrence that weakens the bonds and feelings of belonging to a group threatens the person and may push him to end his life.

Despite the figures that indicate that the suicide rate is high in older persons, many suicides probably occur that do not fit the legal description of the act. When under severe stress, many elderly persons seem to will their own death by refusal to eat, neglect of self-preservation by seclusion, or other methods. Some lives depend upon regular medication or other treatments. Diabetics neglect insulin or other hypoglycemic agents, cardiac medications are neglected, or a variety of other omissions are made. These covert behaviors are difficult to prove, so the true statistics are inaccurate.

Suicide in the elderly is twice as common as in the remainder of the population. Elderly men commit suicide three times more frequently than do women. Suicide is less frequent in elderly married couples, and increases in the single, widowed, and divorced. The suicidal methods attempted by elderly adults are more violent than those of younger persons, which probably indicates that the action is not a play for sympathy and attention, but is a real wish to die.

Elderly persons seldom seek psychiatric or mental health assistance when suicide is contemplated. This may be due to many reasons, such as lack of information about availability, cost, or lack of belief that any help will change their pain of loss. In institutions, the possibility of suicide may not be fully understood nor its danger signs realized, as depression may come to be accepted as normal. Suicide in the elderly has not been studied nor investigated as has suicide in other age groups, and few seem interested in this aspect of death in the elderly.

Tina Matthews was a seventy-year-old woman who had a long and happy married life. John Matthews was a devoted husband, who was a sports editor of a large metropolitan newspaper for many years. Both were avid golfers and because they had no children, they played hard and lived active social lives. As the years advanced, both used beauty aids, massage, vitamins, and every means available to retain youth. As John reached mandatory retirement age, his job was very taxing on him, and he struggled to maintain supremacy. A sudden massive heart attack killed him, and Tina was left at 62 with an expensive home, unpaid for, and a little savings. Advice from lawyers to sell the home, the car, and a mountain cabin and invest the money was acknowledged as the sensible thing to do.

Friends who called and golfing companions eventually lost interest when Tina did not respond. The months passed and Tina's savings dwindled, as had her friends. Then a slight stroke left her with a hesitant step and various aches and pains. Her appearance deteriorated greatly and she saw all that had seemed important in life disappear, never to return. Isolated in her own home, she had no one to talk to and no desire to fight any longer.

Closing the windows and locking the doors, with the oven open and all burners on, she barricaded herself in the kitchen. She was not found for over a week. Doctors, neighbors, friends, grocers, and the paper boy knew she was greatly depressed and had isolated herself. She had spoken frequently of "joining John." When questioned, not one of her contacts felt a woman of her age would do anything to end her life.

Some patients who attempt suicide may be overlooked as potential suicides because they are terminally ill. Persons who have always maintained control over their lives, who have "called their own shots," want control to the end, and to die on their own terms. They tend to plan well, and their attempts are more often than not successful. Terminally ill persons who fear severe pain with fear of losing control of self, are also potential suicides.

When elderly adults are depressed, how does one evaluate their suicide potential? The following factors, if carefully observed, will help determine whether the patient is in danger.

1. Is the person deeply depressed? This is usually a period of inability to plan or act. Has the person been deeply depressed, but now seems improved and more aware and alert to people and surroundings? This is the dangerous time and one of high risk.

2. Is this depression one of a normal reaction to a crisis, or a series of crises, or is it a true psychosis? In psychosis, the person hears voices and they may reveal that he should kill himself and may tell him how. This person is a high risk.

3. Has the patient attempted suicide previously? Was it a serious attempt? Previous serious attempts should be taken as indicators that an attempt may be repeated. If the person talks about dying and reveals he feels suicide is his only choice or that he has thought about suicide, he must be considered a high risk.

4. The nurse may also observe a disturbance in the person's sleep pattern, with early awakening (3:00–7:00 A.M.) in a deep mood of depression.

5. The person may have recently given away articles that were prized and not ordinarily casually exchanged.

6. Nursing personnel familiar with the patient may be unable to describe any particular change in the person but feel "something is wrong, but I can't tell you what it is."

7. Does the depressed person have any support available from others? If the person is a single male without supportive others, the risk is also higher.

If any of these factors or combination of factors are present, help must be obtained rapidly.

The physician will usually prescribe an antidepressant medication immediately. If the patient is not institutionalized, some concerned person must ensure his compliance with the drugs prescribed.

Ideally, psychotherapy should then be given. If the person in danger of suicide is at home, mental health clinics, crisis centers, or private psychologists or psychiatrists may give assistance.

Electroconvulsive therapy (ECT) may be the treatment of choice. Despite its unpopularity, it is used by some physicians, often with excellent results. The resultant short-term memory loss is a decided disadvantage that does not occur with treatment by medication.

Obtaining psychiatric assistance for patients in long-term facilities is almost impossible, unless the patients are paying their own fees. As a result, the care of the depressed, possibly suicidal, elderly adult in a nursing home becomes almost solely a nursing responsibility, and creativity and patience must be used to overcome what may be long-standing behavior.

The patient who has withdrawn and may have suicidal tendencies needs to establish trust with someone. At this stage, the fewer persons involved, the more chance of good rapport. At least one nurse should set aside enough time each day to demonstrate sincere interest in the depressed person. Since these patients demonstrate low self-esteem and are unable to recognize and/or accept the events that precipitated the depression, the following nursing directions will be of assistance in helping the patient to recognize and accept the causes of his depression and improve his self-image.

1. The establishment of rapport and trust are necessary so the patient feels free to discuss his problems.
2. Explore with the patient the events that made former coping mechanisms impossible. Empathetic listening to long-ago events helps the person realize he still has worth.
3. Observe the elderly adult's assets, using sincere praise to reinforce them.
4. Encourage and reinforce a realistic view of the patient's situation (family, environment, health, economics).
5. Encourage the patient to participate in group activities. Do not force choices, at first offer only one possible action. Alternatives can be offered after some improvement in behavior has been observed.
6. If family members are available, assist them to understand the patient's behavior and seek their cooperation.

7. If family members seem to be part of the patient's problem, do not discourage their visits, but try to help them understand each other and assist them in keeping communication open.

When there is any question of suicidal tendences, it is necessary to take special precautions to maintain a safe environment. Long-term care facilities should always be environmentally safe; however, a patient determined to die can be clever in seeking methods. Wandering away from the building to areas of heavy traffic is a quite common method. In the desert Southwest, patients have been observed attempting suicide by wandering away during the summer months, when temperatures often exceed 110°; in such circumstances, death from dehydration would occur within 6–10 hours in the elderly patient. Search and rescue, police, and fire departments are alerted in searches for straying patients. At least one case of depression was cured after an elderly man attempted suicide by the runaway route several times. The frantic attention he received each time convinced him that people did care, that he was worthy of their esteem, and perhaps life was worth living.

Medications are often used to attempt suicide, even when nursing personnel control the drugs. Medication not swallowed can be hoarded, or seemingly innocuous medications, such as aspirin, can be obtained from visitors or by other methods, and lethal doses can result.

Any method others have used can usually be duplicated by patients, and so patient behavior and speech and the effectiveness of antidepressant medications must be closely observed and necessary steps must be taken to prevent suicide.

MENTAL DISEASES OF THE ELDERLY ADULT

Contrary to popular belief, severe mental illness occurs in less than 10 percent of the over-65-years-of-age population. However, as the elderly population increases, the incidence of mental illnesses figure will also rise. Institutional care for mental illness already places a great strain on the health and welfare budgets.

The most common diagnosis of mental illness that the nurse encounters in an institution are "acute brain syndrome" and "chronic brain syndrome." The differentiation between these syndromes and depression—a functional problem—is important in the care of the patient.

The patient may first come to the attention of the physician when his family, landlord, or friends bring him to the office with reports of confusion, disorientation, memory loss, and dementia. These symptoms, which may occur in persons of any age, are more common in the elderly adult. If diagnosis is made solely upon these symptoms of a neuropsychiatric condition, the patient may be released to home or institutional care without any attempt to treat the condition in a belief that it is a sad but anticipated experience in the normal aging process.

Recent studies have shown that persons with moderate-to-severe "chronic brain syndromes" can benefit from sensory stimulation and group therapy. Research is not complete, but ideally, psychiatric therapy should be available.

Acute Brain Syndrome (Nonpsychotic Organic Brain Syndrome)

Patrick Highhouse, a rancher, rode his horse, mended fences, set out cattle salt, and square danced on Saturday night despite his 75 years. Last week he had not returned to the ranch by 6:30 P.M. A search, instigated by his wife, found Pat twenty miles away leading his horse. Inquiry resulted in Pat being unable to remember what he was supposed to be doing and unable to find his way home in the area where he had lived for sixty years. A weekend of rest did not improve the rancher's memory; he spoke less and seemed content to just sit, contrary to his usual vigorous habits. Monday, after a painstaking examination, the physician found that Pat had suffered a myocardial infarction, although no pain was present.

The clue that indicates the presence of acute brain syndrome, rather than other types of mental illness, is the sudden rapid onset of symptoms of mental disorders. The patient has been mentally clear until a short time previous to the problem. The mental disabilities that occur may also be due to such problems as pneumonia, hypoglycemia or hypokalemia, dehydration, painless pulmonary infarction, mild stroke, or drug toxicities.

The treatment of these medical problems by the usual methods results in a gradual reversal of the mental dysfunction as the general health of the patient is improved. This clearing of mental confusion following acute illness of patients in the general hospital is quite frequent in the elderly adult as well as in younger patients.

Chronic Brain Syndrome (Psychosis)

In comparison to acute brain syndrome, which has a sudden onset and is reversible, chronic brain syndrome, which has many similar symptoms, has a gradual onset of six months or longer and is irreversible. Chronic brain syndrome is also known as *organic dementia.* Dementia is an organic loss of intellectual and cognitive function. Orgganic dementia has a variety of forms. The major and most common are arteriosclerotic dementia and Alzheimer's disease.

Alzheimer's Disease (Primary Senile Dementia)

Alzheimer's disease is characterized by progressive deficiencies in understanding, memory, and judgment. The disease begins in the forties and fifties, and the etiology is unknown. Microscopic brain changes, including tangles of neurofibrils, amyloid placques, and pigmentation are found upon brain autopsy, but these are also present in normal findings, although the number of placques seem to determine the presence of abnormal symptoms. The diagnosis can be made by pneumoencephlogram, but computerized tomography is more accurate and is a safer method.

These patients are anxious, aggressive, and compulsive. Memory defects are so severe that daily orientation to the living area may be necessary. This memory defect causes many problems, as the patients are active. As the disease progresses, gait problems increase and convulsions may occur. With time, the patient becomes helpless and requires complete bed care.

Arteriosclerotic Dementia

The arteriosclerotic form of dementia occurs following recurrent cerebrovascular accidents. Cerebral infarction with cerebral softening must be present for dementia to occur. Arteriosclerosis may be present in other areas of the body but need not be found for personality changes to occur.

The patient with arteriosclerotic dementia usually has a residual of neurologic changes following a stroke, depending upon its severity. In addition, after the repeated strokes, the patient will have poor emotional control, characterized by periods of laughing, weeping, and depression. Fatigue, loss of initiative, and shortened attention spans are also present. Suspicion, irritability, and forgetfulness progress to marked confusion, disorientation, incoherence, and other psychotic behaviors. In some persons, severe hostility, criminal acts, and suicide attempts are part of the dementia.

In the past persons diagnosed as having organic brain syndromes (OBS) were institutionalized if the condition was severe and remained institutionalized for life. With the use of various tranquilizers to reduce combativeness and other undesirable behaviors, the person can now live at home or in a day-care facility or a nursing home. A small number of persons do not respond to medication and must be housed in a more protected facility.

Although various psychotropic drugs are valuable in the management of OBS patients, there is danger of oversedation. The activity of the patient will decrease, with danger of pressure sores, pneumonia, malnutrition, and dehydration.

Regardless of how the elderly adult is cared for, the strain on the spouse or family is severe. The loss of the familiar personality of a loved one is traumatic, and feelings of anger, grieving, and guilt must be handled. If the person is to remain at home, some assistance will probably be required, particularly if only an elderly spouse is to be responsible.

Regardless of where the OBS patient is cared for, the environment must be constantly surveyed for safety factors. Potential weapons must be removed and any harmful medications locked up. Vigilance is necessary to prevent roaming, as the patient may be injured and may be a potential danger to others.

Nursing Management

Physical care for OBS patients does not differ greatly from that of other elderly adults, except in degree. The confused state that exists in varying degrees in these patients makes a precise, orderly pattern of daily living easier for them to cope with. Nursing personnel should be familiar to the patient, and care must be taken when new persons are assigned. Routine times for bathing, dressing, eating, toileting, and resting help them maintain regular habits. Specific times for recreational activities need to be included, as the patient must be kept stimulated. This routine should be arrived at with the assistance of the patient rather than dictated to him, if at all possible.

The confused adult needs to be constantly reoriented. If he makes errors about where he is, or about the time, date, or other facts, it is not a kindness to agree or to ignore the error. He must be corrected in a matter-of-fact manner that is not judgmental. A profusion of calendars, clocks, directional signs, and announcements of diversional activities will be of assistance in the facility. Addressing the patient directly, always using his name, and reminding the patient of the nurse's name is also helpful in maintaining orientation. Any illusions, that is, the misinterpretations of the real identity of an object, must be corrected.

Joe Mills was up and dressed by 5:30 A.M. each morning, as he has been for thirty years of the day shift in a steel mill. At 82, as a resident in a long-term care facility, he sat on a bench waiting till a night nurse had time to give him a cup of coffee.

A new housekeeping routine meant that Frank, a maintenance man, polished the floors with a heavy electric buffer that he slowly swung from side to side. Later in the day, Joe Mills related to his nurse how Frank looked for money with a metal detector on the floor each morning.

His nurse used the correct method of dealing with illusions: (1) she listened carefully to Joe's recital of the facts; (2) she did not contradict the story, but stated that it did not seem correct to her; (3) she investigated and found the reality; (4) she took Joe to see the polisher, explained its use and why he had not seen it before and alerted Frank to talk to Joe the next morning when he polished.

Illusions are only one example of loss of reality. Patients must be reoriented to person, place, and time to prevent further agitation. When reorienting, touch the patient, establish eye contact, and speak slowly and clearly. Orientation must be constantly repeated until the patient is no longer confused.

The confused patient must understand what is expected of him as consistent behavior. Disruptive behavior in the elderly adult is not uncommon. Limitations can be placed upon behavior.

Each morning when a male student practical nurse went into Alex Zarkny's room, Alex swore at him and threw anything available. As a result, Mrs. Grant always volunteered to bathe Alex, as she could "handle" him. Alex's behavior rewarded him by getting just what he wanted.

After a nursing conference that identified the problem, the personnel agreed on a consistent approach. If a nurse was rejected, Alex would be told that no one would care for him other than bring his food tray and water until he accepted the assigned caretaker. Mrs. Grant would not be assigned. A nurse approached four times on two shifts and offered care and was rejected by the patient. The next day, the student offered his help and was accepted; no further problems with nursing favorites were encountered.

Any limitation placed upon behavior must be done by the consistent approach of all personnel, preferably as a result of group problem solving. The patient must never be rejected, only his behavior. Praise for cooperation, with generous use of touch, listening to the patient or walking with him, will also reward the behavioral modification. Success is not instantaneous, and consistency may be difficult. Not all behaviors can be changed; some must simply be endured. Later attempts may be more successful. Personnel must resist the temptation to punish aggravating behavior by words or other methods. This type of reaction by staff rewards the patient, and the behavior will be repeated.

When disruptive behavior is modified, the result is rewarding because care of the patient is easier and the atmosphere more liveable, for both nurses and patients.

REVIEW QUESTIONS

1. Define *crisis* and list several crises common to the elderly adult.
2. Describe behaviors that may be observed in the anxious patient.
3. Explain a physical reason for depression and its causes.
4. Give one explanation of why suicide rates for elderly adults may be incorrect.
5. When is the danger of suicide the greatest?
6. Which of the organic brain syndromes is reversible and why?

BIBLIOGRAPHY

Bellak, Leopold. *The Best Years of Your Life*. New York: Atheneum, 1975.

Bureau of Census: *Statistical Abstracts of the United States* 1975. Washington, D.C.: U.S. Government Printing Office, 1975.

Burnside, Irene Mortenson. "Reality Testing: An Important Concept." *Association of Rehabilitation Nurses* 2 (May/June 1977): 3-4, 6-7, 9.

Ernst, Philip, et al. "Treatment of the Aged Mentally Ill. Further Unmasking of the Effects of Diagnosis of Chronic Brain Syndrome." *Journal of the American Geriatric Society* 25 (October 1977): 466-469.

Friedman, Joyce S. "Cry for Help: Suicide in the Aged." *Journal of Gerontological Nursing*. 2 (May/June 1976): 28-32.

––––––– . "Nurse Specialist Uses Reminiscing Therapy with the Elderly." *American Journal of Nursing* 78 (November 1978): 1958.

Kopell, Bert S. "Treating the Suicidal Patient." *Geriatrics* 32 (September 1977): 65-67.

MacDonald, Larry. "Behavioral Therapy: Its Application to Reduce Disruptive Behaviors of the Elderly in Nursing Homes." *The Canadian Nurse* 73 (July 1977): pp. 26-29.

Milt, Harry. *Basic Handbook on Mental Illness*, 3d ed. Maplewood, N.J.: Scientific Aids Publications, 1976.

National Center for Health Statistics of the United States, *Vol. II, Mortality, Part A*. Washington, D.C.: U.S. Government Printing Office, 1975.

Oberleder, Muriel. "Managing Problem Behaviors of Elderly Patients." *Hospital and Community Psychiatry* 27 (May 1976): 325-330.

Reichel, William. "Organic Brain Syndromes in the Aged." *Hospital Practice* 7 (May 1976): 119-125.

Selye, Hans. "A Code for Coping with Stress." *AORN Journal* 25 (January 1977): 35-42.

Teeter, Ruth, et al. "Psychiatric Disturbances of Aged Patients in Skilled Nursing Homes." *The American Journal of Psychiatry* 12 (December 1976): 1430-1433.

––––––– . "Nursing Aspects in the Care of the Elderly." *Nursing Times* 74 (April 1978): 626-629.

chapter 4

Social-Psychological Needs
of the Elderly

OBJECTIVES

After studying this unit, the student will be able to:

1. Describe some of the needs of patients' families when they place a relative in a long-term care facility.

2. Describe some patient behaviors that are nonverbal methods of expressing the need for love.

3. List some ways in which residency in a long-term care facility can reduce self-esteem or respect.

4. Discuss the goals of a diversional activity program in a long-term care facility.

5. Identify the nurse's responsibility for the success of diversional activities.

6. Describe several ways that nurses can assist the patient in meeting his spiritual needs.

ASSISTING WITH THE SOCIAL AND EMOTIONAL NEEDS OF THE ELDERLY ADULT

Suffering is not unique to the elderly adult, but this age group's physical, emotional, and economic problems are usually greater than those of other segments of the population.

If physical illness is present, emotional problems may also be found. The multiple stresses on the elderly may cause increased problems in mental health. The elderly person's whole reality of life may be made up of unpleasant facts.

Some of the sources of suffering by the elderly adults are as follows:

- Illness is usually common and complex, and reoccurs frequently. The loss of mastery over one's body, the changes in self-image, and the independence that a strong functioning body gives are lost, and self-esteem is greatly diminished.

- Emotional trauma may be caused by the imagined or actual attitude of physicians and other health professionals in turning away from the person. The message that "nothing further can be done" or that he is being belittled is received by the person. Self-respect is damaged as one feels lack of worth, status, and prestige.

- Family, relatives, and friends are lost by death, separation, or estrangement. These events reduce the elderly person's sense of belonging and the sources of giving and receiving love. Beloved possessions are gradually discarded, given away, or worn out. The close association of these objects with the people who gave them, shared them, and used them is akin to loss of love and further reduces a sense of belonging.

These and other causes of suffering are present in each person who is admitted to a nursing home. The elderly adult may emerge from these traumatic events with ego intact, but those who are less able to cope may have feelings of inadequacy, insecurity, loneliness, and isolation. The basic needs for love, belonging, self-esteem, and self-respect have been reduced or lost.

Nursing personnel are not only caretakers of the body, but of the whole person. The personnel of the institution become the surrogate family of the residents. They must take every measure possible

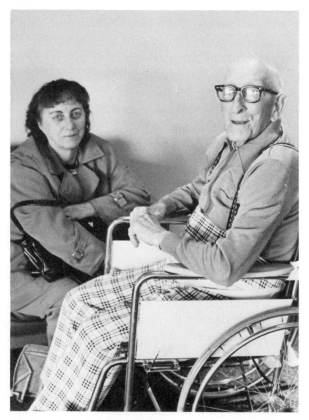

Photographer: Doris Wilson, RN
Models: George Snyder, Hazel Thomas

Family members and visitors play an important part in the adjustment of the elderly adult.

to assist the elderly person to adapt to his new life. Any actions that the nurse takes to help the patients retain or regain their independence will enhance their confidence. Her recognition of the person as an individual will bolster self-esteem and self-respect.

Family

Relatives, friends, and family are probably the most important factors in the patient's life. Therefore, the nurse's attitude toward the family is as important as is her attitude toward the patient.

When a parent or relative must be placed in a long-term care facility, the family usually feels guilty about their actions. They often need to give repeated explanations to nursing personnel of why this was necessary. If they are not helped, the result may be that they cease or reduce their visits. The nurse can explain that guilt is a common result of placement, but emphasize that it was a joint decision with the doctor (and, it is hoped, with the patient), and was done with best of motives. Listening in a nonjudgmental manner as long as is necessary for the family is the most beneficial action the nurse can take.

The nurse's support, and her attitude of concern for the patient will reduce the family's anxiety and fear. The nurse's acceptance of the family will help to reduce the patient's feeling of loneliness. Cordial relations with nursing staff help establish positive relationships and stimulate further interactions between patient and family.

Love

The need for love is difficult to define. Sexual love is only one part of the larger emotion. The person needs to feel that someone has a deep, calm, enduring emotional regard for him.

The lack of love may not be realized on a conscious basis, but the behavior of a patient reaching out for emotional support can be readily observed.

Mamie Shaw was alone. No visitors came to see her—she had outlived friends and relatives. Nursing personnel cared for her as quickly as possible, as each encounter with her resulted in constant complaints—her head hurt, her food sat in her stomach, her knees ached. Sudden outbursts of anger directed at anyone in sight caused reciprocal behavior in nursing personnel. Despite demands for all types of services, their delivery did not result in satisfaction, and Mamie's call light was frequently on.

This type of behavior is not uncommon. Crying, reaching out for people, increased eating and talking are nonverbal mannerisms that give evidence of need.

Mamie's behavior changed gradually after nurses decided that their behavior must also change. As a result of a problem-solving conference, the nurses decided to (1) acknowledge their understanding of her anger, at the same time putting an arm about her shoulder if possible; (2) give care in a relaxed manner, spending as much time as possible with her, which was not as the result of her demands; (3) give special attention to her grooming and praising her frequently; (4) regardless of provocation, refrain from arguing and attempt to establish better communications; (5) encourage Mamie to enter into conversation with other residents.

Elderly adults often question nurses about their behavior: Why am I angry? Why do I cry easily? Why do I complain so much? Some see this behavior as a sign of "senility" or mental disease. The nurse can explain that being away from family and friends reduces the amount of love and attention that we need. The patients should be reassured that their feelings are normal for the situation and that other persons feel the same.

The patient's somatic complaints that cannot be diagnosed should not be ridiculed nor attributed to psychological causes. The nurse's refusal to accept the complaint will increase the patient's anxiety. These complaints should be seen as hints that nonphysical problems are present. The nurse can give assistance and attention to the complaints by giving back rubs, attending to comfortable surroundings, and by listening and communicating to learn the reasons for the body ailments. Consistent words of kindness, the use of touch, and general respect will help decrease the need for somatic complaints.

During any period of emotional upset, the natural inclination of the nurse is to attempt to discover the cause. These attempts must not be so vigorous that the person is forced into discussing a topic that is emotionally painful and that results in highly charged responses and increased anxiety. Any conversation that results in increased anxiety should be quickly refocused by the nurse into safer topics. Patients have the right to mental as well as physical privacy. They have a right to refuse to discuss feelings until they feel that sharing them will result in comfort and reduction of anxiety.

In the process of reaching out for attention and love, some patients use actions that are unacceptable, such as pinching or squeezing. They must be told their actions are not acceptable. If the patient understands that this is not a rejection and that specific time will be spent with him, and if efforts are made to show attention and regard, the behavior can usually be reversed.

Retaining Self-respect and Self-esteem

The multiple stresses that the elderly adult suffers may result in loss of self-respect and self-esteem. The nurse must be alert to avoid any actions or behaviors that may cause further losses. The way in which elderly adults regard themselves is the key to their happiness and their ability to adapt to life.

Privacy

One of the drawbacks of any communal living arrangement is the loss of privacy. Many long-term care facilities have no private rooms. If there are private rooms, they may be reserved for the more seriously ill or have other restrictions on their use. The patient may share a room with one other person or a number of persons.

Our society values a certain amount of personal space—enough to maintain personal privacy. Possession of this space results in feelings of security; loss of the space will result in anxiety. For example, being surrounded by dense crowds at a sporting event will prove disturbing to most people. This condition does not last long and can be tolerated, because it will change. However, living under conditions in which privacy is impossible and is constantly invaded without one's permission results in loss of competence to control one's life. Privacy is essential to competence: one needs to be able to decide when one wishes to be alone or when to be with others. Privacy is also required as a retreat from painful, anxiety-producing, situations.

Nurses must exercise care that the patient's rights to privacy are always respected. The living area of his bedroom should be respected in the same manner as if it were his private living area at home. If the room has double or multiple occupancy, cubicle curtains must be provided. If the curtains are drawn, permission to enter must be asked. Closets and drawers must also be respected as private property. It is, however, necessary to clean these areas for some patients and in such cases prior permission should be sought. Entry should be demanded only if there is adequate reason to believe that the private areas contain something of danger to the patient or others.

All treatments should be performed in privacy, and the patient should be adequately draped if he is removed from his room for bathing. Exposure to persons other than the caretaker is humiliating and lowers one's self-respect. When the nurse is working alone with the patient, she must also take care that the patient is not unduly exposed. The permissive mores of today's generation are not those of the older generation. Modesty is valued; it is a habit of long standing that must be respected.

The patient's clothing and possessions should be treated with care and marked for identification if necessary. Their use should never be shared with other patients, unless the patient has so requested.

Nurses should avoid any actions or words that will cause embarrassment to the patient. The discussion of any of the person's problems, or comments about him or his family in the presence of other patients will cause the patient to feel he can no longer cope with life's situations since they are common knowledge and may result in ridicule by others.

Use of Names

The use of one's full name and title reflects the respect of the person speaking. Most persons outside your family and circle of friends address you by your full name. Informality is prevalent in society today, particularly among younger people. Elderly adults were raised in an era of more formality, and should be addressed as Mrs. Smith, Mr. Jones, or Miss Green, unless they have specifically requested that their given names be used.

Greeting the elderly adult as "Granny," "Gramps," "Aunty" or other such terms, is demeaning. Regardless of the fact that the patient may not complain, the nurse should not address nor allow others to address the person in this manner. Names are one of the few possessions peculiarly our own, and their recognition by others helps us to retain our self-esteem.

Belonging

Belonging is a basic need of life. Our relationships with others are important throughout our lives. As we age, these relationships seem to become more important, and part of our contentment and

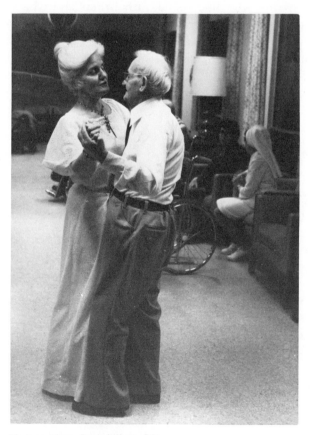

Photographer: Doris Wilson, RN
Models: Dr. Earl Drum, Bernadine Redwine

Belonging and loving.

satisfaction in life may depend upon friendships. A friend who can be confided in is helpful to the mental health of the confider. The multiple crises of the elderly adult can be tolerated and dealt with more effectively if he has a trusted confidant.

Some persons are more likely to have confidants than others. Husbands tend to confide in wives, but the wife is more apt to confide in a child. Neither is likely to confide in his siblings.

No specific study has been done on the confidants of persons living in long-term care facilities. If there are a great number of opportunities for interaction among the residents, it seems likely that friendships that promote the trust necessary for confidences will occur. Many factors—such as length of residence, mobility, and general health—will affect the formation of relationships.

The patients who like to be with others and who have in the past had confidants are the most likely to again form these relationships. The nurse is always available and seems to be greatly utilized as a confidant. Each patient should have someone, either a nurse, a friend, a relative, or a spiritual adviser, in whom he can confide.

Patient Government

Many long-term care facilities have patient government organizations. The structure is usually simple; one person is elected as chairman, and rarely are other officers used. The residents meet one a week or more often, and have a number of possible functions such as (1) listening to complaints and discussion of them, and forwarding those that seem valid to administration; (2) helping to plan activities; (3) welcoming and assisting in the orientation of new residents; and (4) requesting changes, and making suggestions to the administration.

A great deal of the success of the government and the continued interest in it by the residents depends upon the leader. Leadership also changes frequently, so the group may fluctuate.

The group meetings and decision making activities are helpful in promoting a feeling of some mastery over life and a feeling of belonging.

One active group sent representatives to the local Senior Center meetings and to Council on Aging legislative hearings. Another group has a "work" committee, which contracts for such jobs as addressing and stuffing envelopes, packaging sample giveaways, quilting, and tying quilts. The money they earn is used for parties, outings, and equipment. They also volunteer to do similar tasks for service organizations. These small contributions help the patients more than the recipients of the service. Confidence, pride, recognition, and attention contribute to positive mental health.

In assisting with emotional needs, if the patient can derive satisfaction from his relationship with family, fellow residents, and nursing personnel, he will be less likely to focus on his health and body. A trusted confidant, kindness, and loving touches will do much to alleviate emotional suffering.

The nurse must be mature enough emotionally and have her own sources of emotional satisfaction in order to be able to give the support necessary to patients without expecting to receive it in return.

ASSISTING WITH THE SPIRITUAL NEEDS OF THE PATIENT

Throughout the history of man, both early and civilized, he has been seeking the guidance and assistance of a divine being. Our present society has been labeled by some as irreligionist, immoral, and sinful. A recent trend, particularly popular with some groups of young people, has been to put less emphasis on material success and more on developing spiritual strengths. Ethics, brotherly love, and faith are more important to these young people than individual religious doctrine.

The religion of the elderly adult, at present, tends to be more formalized, and makes certain demands upon its followers. The patient must be able to satisfy his spiritual needs during his residency in the long-term care facility, as religion is part of his value system and plays an important part in our individual lives and in our entire society. Many people report that religion seems more important to them during the last years of their lives than at any other time in their lives. Many persons never had the opportunity during the early years of their lives, when they were busy with jobs, children, and homes, to devote as much time as they would have liked to their religion. For elderly adults, the retirement years provide the perfect opportunity to develop spiritually and to sort out their past.

Nurses probably reflect the level of knowledge of the majority of our population: they know only about the religion that they and/or their families endorse. If one has had the privilege of travel and observed or participated in religious celebrations other than

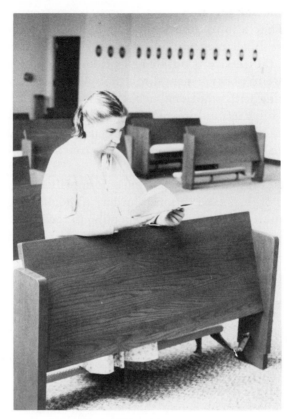

Photographer: Doris Wilson, RN
Model: Angeline Weinoda

Worship is an integral part of life for many elderly adults.

one's own, or studied other religions, it is easier to relate to others' beliefs. It is only necessary, however, to accept the commonalities of all religions—that is, belief in a supreme being, force, or code—to respect other ways of expression.

If the nurse believes that each person is an individual and must be cared for in a manner that preserves his uniqueness, then religious conviction or lack of it will be seen as another facet of the patient's total personality. The nurses' responsibility for comprehensive care includes assisting the patient to meet these spiritual needs. The three major components of these needs may be identified as religion, faith, and worship.

Religion is the belief in a divine or superhuman power, which is worshipped and obeyed. It is also a specific set of beliefs and practies. To be religious does not necessitate membership in a specific body of worshipers: religion may simply be a personal commitment.

If the patient requests that his religious adviser be called, the nurse should attend to the call promptly, When such an adviser visits, he should be met with proper respect, and the privacy of the meeting should be protected. If assistance or articles for administration of sacraments are required, provide them or have them available before the minister arrives.

If the patient requires special dietary modification to meet his religious obligations, these should be thoroughly understood. Family and religious advisers may need to be questioned for a thorough understanding of the specific requirements. The physician must also understand the restriction so that he may weigh his decision on diet orders. The dietary department must be informed because the preparation of special diets is their responsibility. If the dietary observations are not honored, this may cause the patient intense anxiety, guilt, and depression.

The elderly adult may have with him certain religious articles, such as a Bible, Koran, or other book, crucifix, religious medal, rosary, prayer shawl, or other paraphernalia. These belongings represent far more to the patient than other types of belongings: they must be handled with respect, regardless of personal beliefs.

If the long-term facility has religious services, the nurse should make sure that every patient who wishes to attend will have any assistance necessary to insure their presence at the meeting.

Care must also be taken that no patient who does not wish to attend services or receive visits from religious workers or clergymen is ever coerced into doing so. Neither does the nurse have the right to proselytize for her religion.

Worship is church service, prayer, or other practice showing reverence for the almighty. Worship can be private; it need not conform to any specific rite.

At times of stress, or as a routine measure, the patient may request that the nurse pray with him. If you are familiar with the prayer and wish to join in, the meaning to the patient will be intensified; if you do not wish to do so, all that is necessary is an attitude of quiet. If the patient is unable to formulate a prayer and asks for your help, whether or not you are accustomed to praying, you might pray in the same manner you would for your loved ones.

> Lord, help me bear my suffering.
> Lord, I offer you my love.
> Lord, remember me.

Formal prayer is no more than a few sincere phrases.

Reading religious magazines, Bibles, or prayer books for those unable to do so may not seem to be nursing to some persons. Any action that the patient is unable to do for himself and that brings comfort is nursing at its best.

Listening is perhaps the greatest tool that the nurse possesses. She will often find the patient confiding in her. Nursing, as part of its ethical code, has always pledged to serve persons of all races, religions, and creeds and to hold in confidence all personal matters entrusted to them.

Patients will explain their beliefs and discuss their actions at certain times of their lives and ask the nurse for her opinion—the activity is much like a confession with the patient asking for forgiveness.

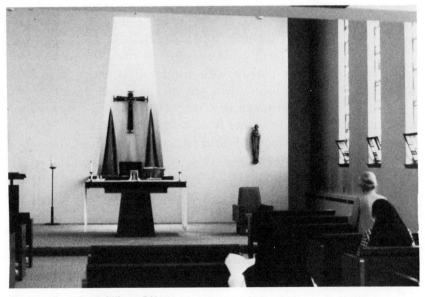

Photographer: Doris Wilson, RN

A quiet place to renew the spirit is essential for patients and families.

The patient may repeat the same conversation to a number of care-takers in a search for comfort. Nurses should not judge the person's actions or his revelations, but should listen with genuine interest and stay with the patient while he prays.

Faith is the absolute trust in the goodness of the diety, the knowledge that God is with you. Faith may also be that specific set of beliefs that is peculiar to a particular religion. The faith of the elderly adult who has had numerous trials in life, who is now ill, per-haps alone in life, is tremendously important. Faith helps to reaffirm the value of life and gives meaning to it.

In caring for the patient who has need for spiritual assistance, the nurse who understands her own philosophy of life and has some religious education will be most at ease. It may be that this area of care is extremely difficult for some nurses because of their own personal needs. Until a nurse can be comfortable enough so that no anxiety is carried to the patient, a substitute nurse may need to be used. Nurses cannot be all things to all people.

PROVIDING DIVERSIONAL ACTIVITIES

Goals and Requirements

The goal of diversional activities in a long-term care facility is to in-volve each resident in one or more activities that will assist in keeping the person mentally, physically, and socially active.

All facilities that are Medicare certified are required to have an activity program that is supervised by an experienced director. The director is responsible for developing a plan for each patient to par-ticipate in independent or group activities.

The long-term care facility must provide sufficient space for the activity program. Areas for crafts, games, exercise sessions, and social gatherings are required. Adequate supplies and equipment must be available for patient's use.

The activity program also requires sufficient personnel for ade-quate planning, record keeping, transportation, and directing the var-ious aspects of the department. The more varied the program and the more patients involved the more staff members are required to meet the goals of the department. Volunteer workers may be used exten-sively, but salaried staff are necessary for the direction and continu-ity of the program.

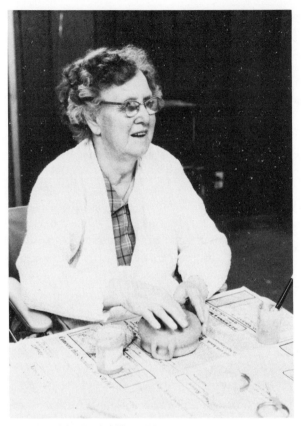

Photographer: Doris Wilson, RN
Model: Signa Lundberg

A blind patient learns the satisfaction of a new skill.

The activity director or one of her personnel interview the patient shortly after admission to the residence. The patient is questioned about his hobbies and skills and what types of activities he enjoys. The activity program is explained to him, and he is invited to participate in it. The director also interviews nursing personnel to discover what the patient's limitations may be, what his strengths are, and if the doctor has indicated that the patient may participate in all activities.

Matching personnel with suitable activities is based upon the patient's needs and interests. If the elderly adult needs to exercise his hands to maintain function, then ceramic projects may be desirable. Macrame might also be helpful, but perhaps the fingers are not agile enough for this to be successful. A patient confined to a wheelchair may need exercise to maintain function and position change, so he will be invited to join the exercise group for daily workouts. A patient unable to participate in specific activities, who needs to socialize with people, can join a "Chat and Chew" group. Bingo may help keep another patient alert and improve eye-hand coordination.

The activity plan for each patient, arrived at with their participation, is written for departmental use and incorporated into the patient care plan on the nursing unit. Activity program personnel make periodic summaries of the participation of the patient in the activities.

Program Examples

Individual activities are provided for persons who do not care for large group participation. Some participate as helpers and transport those in wheelchairs. One man made his own activity: he sings "Happy Birthday" in his beautifully trained voice to each resident on his day.

The television, radio, and stereophonic equipment can also be used individually to provide a great deal of entertainment. The placement of television sets in the patients' rooms remains controversial: it may cause further seclusion and should only be used by bed patients. Communal sets do force more interaction, and probably are

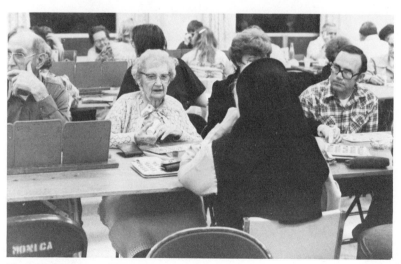

Photographer: Doris Wilson, RN
Model: Minnie Cull

Bingo helps this patient's concentration and improves eye-hand coordination.

less disturbing to others because they are placed in dayrooms and lounges.

Activities outside the residence are valuable because they provide variety and stimulus. Picnics are always popular, whether in new settings or on the facility grounds. Horseshoes, croquet, and gossip may help make the day. Music by volunteers always proves to be popular. One church periodically provides their big buses to take patients for a ride. To see how the old neighborhood has changed or to view the world outside helps the patients' orientation to time and place.

Some of the elderly adults are confined to their beds, but simple ceramic projects, knitting, crocheting, or reading help make the days more enjoyable and the boredom or pain less overwhelming. "Talking books"—those recorded for persons with visual problems— are also popular.

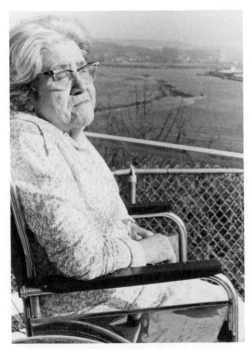

Photographer: Doris Wilson, RN
Model: Fawn Bealer

Surveying the familiar waterfront in the background keeps this woman interested in the outside world.

Participation Difficulties

The goal of diversional activity is to involve all patients. In reality, this is impossible. Some patients are physically or mentally unable to participate. Other patients do not participate for a variety of reasons. When today's elderly adults were active and working, there may have been fewer hours for leisure, less information about hobbies, and less money to spend on nonessential items. There was also a more rigid set of customs about what was suitable for men and what was suitable for women to do. Men who have been employed most of their lives in strenuous jobs such as steel workers, lumber-product workers, or miners find it difficult to be interested in less physical activities. The ability to use leisure time in a mentally and physically therapeutic manner or even to enjoy it is not an American trait.

Women seem to find it easier and more enjoyable to participate in activity programs than men do. Many have always done handwork, and it has been more acceptable for women to have leisure activities. Handwork often provided essential clothing, bedding, and other items for family use and was not really a hobby.

Directors' Problems

Regardless of the value, variety, and interest of the programs planned by the activity department, the director may have poor patient participation. Schedules for the month's activities are usually widely displayed throughout the residence. Nursing personnel must realize the importance of socialization and activity in the life of the elderly adult. Therefore, coordination of treatments, medications, bathing, and dressing must be done so patients are free to attend activities.

When the nurse is interested in the total welfare of the elderly patient, she will encourage him to participate, remind him of the time schedule, and comment upon his involvement. The success of the activity program depends upon the cooperation of all staff members.

The activity director may have detailed plans for a therapeutic program, but she must also have sufficient monies budgeted for adequate supplies, adequate space that is pleasant and comfortable, and enough staff to carry out the plan.

Diversional activities that stimulate the mind and provide for physical activity are as important as the physical care of the patient in maintaining a positive attitude toward life.

REVIEW QUESTIONS

1. List three reasons why it is important to have good rapport with the patient's family.
2. Explain why it is important to respect the privacy of the patient.
3. The patient has a number of somatic complaints each day. List some nursing measures that may help reduce this behavior.
4. Explain the goals of a diversional activity program.
5. The patient is unable to leave his bed and relates his past interest in his church. Describe how the nurse may assist.

BIBLIOGRAPHY

Aguilera, Donna C. *Crisis Intervention.* St. Louis: C. V. Mosby, 1974.

Blondis, Marion Nebbett, and Barbara E. Jackson. *Non-Verbal Communication with Patients; Back to Human Touch.* New York: A Wiley Medical Publication, 1977.

Burnside, I. M. "Recognizing and Reducing Emotional Problems in the Aged. *Nursing '77* 7 (March 1977): 56-59.

Dickinson, Sister Corita. "The Search for Spiritual Meaning." *American Journal of Nursing.* 75 (October 1975): 1789.

Fox, N. L. "Nursing Intervention: Holiday Happiness—All Year 'Round. How to put Joy into Geriatric Care." *Journal of Practical Nursing* 28 (December 1978): 20-22.

Henderson, Virginia, and Gladys Nite. *Principles and Practice of Nursing,* 6th ed. New York: Macmillan, 1978, pp. 1018-1054.

Hoff, Lee Ann. *People in Crisis, Understanding and Helping.* Menlo Park, Calif.: Addison-Wesley Publishing Co., 1978.

Hubert, Sister Mary. "Spiritual Care for Every Patient." *The Journal of Nursing Education* 2 (May/June 1963): 9-11.

Maslow, Abraham. *Motivation and Personality.* New York: Harper and Brothers, 1954.

Morris, Karen, and John Foerster. "Team Work: Nurse and Chaplain." *American Journal of Nursing* 75 (October 1975): 1789.

Papalea, Deane E., and Sally W. Olds. *Human Development.* New York: McGraw-Hill, 1978.

Roberts, Sharon L. *Behavioral Concepts and the Critically Ill Patient.* Englewood Cliffs, N.J.: Prentice-Hall, Inc., 1976.

Saxton, Dolores F., and Phyllis Haring. *Care of Patients with Emotional Problems.* St. Louis: C. V. Mosby Co., 1975.

Shontz, Franklin. *The Psychological Aspects of Physical Illness and Disability.* New York: Macmillan, 1975.

Vaillot, Sister Madeline Clemence. "The Spiritual Factors in Nursing." *Journal of Practical Nursing* 20 (September, 1970): 30.

Weiner, M. B., et al. "A Psychotherapeutic Approach to Emotional Problems of the Elderly." *Journal of Nursing Care* 11 (May 1978): 14–15.

―――――. "Grandpa or grand person . . . do we really care?" *Nursing Times* 74 (October 5, 1978): 1626–1627.

The Final Cycle of Life

OBJECTIVES

After studying this unit, the student will be able to:

1. Discuss how mandatory retirement may change life patterns.

2. List some of the plans for life that should be made prior to retirement.

3. Describe some alterations in work patterns that may decrease the trauma of retirement.

4. List several methods of care, other than physical, that will help to comfort the dying patient.

5. Describe several ways that other patients and relatives may be of assistance to the dying person.

6. Discuss why the dying should not be isolated and how people may unconsciously isolate them.

RETIREMENT

Retirement is one of the major crises faced by people in our society. Despite the fact that a sizable portion of our population is publically supported, the philosophy of our culture is basically work-oriented.

Our lives are centered about our jobs: our work hours, vacations, and standard of living are dictated by our jobs. Frequently, the majority of our social contacts are provided by job-related associates. Our recreation may also be centered there, with team sports or recreational centers sponsored by the company. Our health care may also be dictated by the union contract under which we work or by the company's fringe benefit package.

Small wonder, then, that when our employment ceases, our income, health care, and recreational and social lives are changed. Planning for successful retirement must begin long before the actual day of retirement. Planning for future income is imperative. The amount one will receive as a result of Social Security income can be closely estimated years in advance, as can company pensions. Adequate income for the future is one basis of successful retirement. Unfortunately, regardless of planning, some people are unable to acquire additional funds and must depend solely on Social Security benefits.

Retirement Planning

Persons who planned for their retirement ten years or more in advance, and who had been able to save enough to comfortably augment their pensions, may find—because of inflation, inaccurate or unrealistic planning for the number of years they would survive, or because major illnesses were not foreseen—that their savings are now exhausted. In saving for retirement, the rate of inflation must be allowed for, with no assurance that any given amount will be adequate.

Successful retirement must include some type of stimulating activity that will help fill the void created by freedom from work. At this period of life, few people choose an entirely new interest, although this is not impossible. Activities should be chosen with as much care as a job was chosen in earlier life, because equipment, supplies, lessons, and other considerations may be costly. Certainly one's skills, interest, and abilities must be considered. Activities are even more valuable if they can be used to supplement income. In some instances, they lead to full-time second careers.

A few people may be content to "do nothing" and do not require meaningful activity to be happy. Americans are said to be unable to enjoy leisure, but this is simply conjecture.

The use of leisure time to assist others is probably the most satisfying and fulfilling of all work. The need for volunteers is tremendous. One may work with handicapped children or adults, be a teacher's aide, coach a team of children, be a foster grandparent, or develop an entirely new helping role.

A widespread American dream voiced by many retirees is to travel. Many sell their homes and buy travel trailers or motorhomes. They often find that temporary homes are not their ideal, and that constant movement palls quickly, particularly if travel was not their previous way of life. This type of life is costly and demands a certain level of health. Prior to making any permanent decisions, there should be a trial vacation with rented vehicles. Energy shortages may strictly curtail this type of life in the near future.

The location and type of housing chosen for retirement is one of the deciding factors in contentment. Ideally, staying in the same home or apartment in the location one is accustomed to will result in the greatest satisfaction. Unfortunately, with the prospect of less income, perhaps a less expensive home with lower taxes and maintenance should be considered. The home or apartment may be too large to maintain, or have stairs that are difficult to climb. Many elderly adults, because of lower costs, choose mobile homes. This type of home is convenient and easily managed. Although this may seem to be an advantage, the lack of yard work and the compact surroundings may prove detrimental to the couple's intention to remain active. The lack of space necessary to do many types of hobby work may be another drawback of mobile-home living. The reduction of space may also result in reduction of privacy for the couple. Some area that can be used as a "hideaway" is useful in maintaining harmonious relations when persons are constantly together, as they are in retirement.

Relocation to a new geographic area or to a retirement community seems ideal for many elderly adults. In the process, the familiar home and many treasured possessions are sold. Friends and family members may be left behind in the move. After the initial delight of new surroundings and climate, many people realize that they are unable to adapt to this radical change and are unhappy and depressed. Usually, monetary considerations make it impossible to relocate a second time. It is particularly traumatic if one of the couple dies and the survivor is left in the new location separated from old friends and family.

Final decisions should never be made without a "trial run." Ideally, to further evaluate the wisdom of permanent settlement, a vacation should be spent in the new location during a period when the worst climatic conditions are present.

The same delayed decisions should be used prior to moving in with children, unless there is no alternative. The parent must be flexible and avoid trying to run the household. Parents must not assume the dependent role, where their demands become a type of regression. The successful integration of the parent into the child's home will be easier if there are no grandchildren present. Although harmony is possible, many report that failure of the elderly to bridge the generation gap is a common adjustment problem where grandchildren are present. Efforts to adapt to an elderly parent joining a household must be made by the entire family, and the elderly may prove to be more flexible than their children or grandchildren.

The loss of a longtime spouse by death or divorce during the period when one is also facing the retirement crisis may greatly hinder or prevent adequate adjustment to either or both life changes.

Insurance after Retirement

When an employee retires, his customary health plan ceases, and he must pay his own premiums. Most insurance companies have arrangements whereby the retiring person can retain his health policy, but the payments are higher than those of his former group policy.

Almost all persons over age 65 are covered by Medicare, parts A and B (hospital and medical insurance). Medicare coverage pays approximately 40 percent of medical costs. According to one's financial condition, one may or may not be eligible for Medicaid coverage. The wisest plan is have supplemental insurance that will help cover additional costs.

Informed people everywhere must be aware of the existence of insurance schemes that, although they may be legal, prey on the fears of the older adult. Many persons are not aware of what benefits they have under Medicare and, under pressure from agents who cloud the issue, purchase policies that do not meet their needs, duplicate their present coverage, and threaten their income. Investigation reveals that some of the worst weaknesses of these policies is that some have waiting periods of up to two years before they take effect, and not all payments are 100 percent tax deductible.

Insurance to complement Medicare should include the following conditions: (1) preexisting conditions for the six months immediately preceding the policy should be the only ones affecting denial of payment; (2) set amounts of coverage per day should not be specified, rather a percentage of the total remaining bill should be paid by insurance; and (3) the policy should cover gaps in other insurance policies, and not duplicate what is already available.

The elderly adult should be aware that health programs that assist him outside the institutional setting will not only be less expensive, they will probably also be better for his physical and mental well-being, unless he is seriously ill.

When to Retire

Many Americans have no choice about when to retire—they must work as long as possible because of their financial situation. Many persons would prefer to retire at 65 years or before. Monetarily, many would be in a more favorable tax situation and would actually be as well off, or better, living on their pensions, which are largely tax free. More time to spend in pursuit of their own interests may be more attractive than job and money. The oft-heard story of persons who do not survive long after retirement at 65–70 years may be an additional inducement to retire as early as possible in an effort to

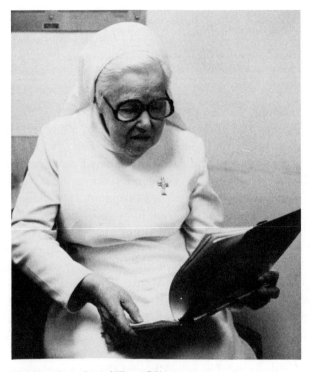

Photographer: Doris Wilson, RN
Model: Sister M. Fabian

This registered nurse works several hours each week—even though past normal retirement age.

add additional years to a work-free later life. Only about 25 percent of retirement-age persons rate their health as "poor," and this is not as common a reason for retirement as is usually believed.

With the new mandatory age for retirement extended to 70 years for many occupations, it will take several years to ascertain whether there is a trend toward staying longer on the job. For many, the years between ages 65 and 70 will be characterized by the increased effort necessary to produce a satisfactory work load. The quality of work and the intellect necessary to produce do not change, but the muscular and mental reactions do slow down. Ideally, the later working years should be ones of gradual slowing down, where either fewer days per week or fewer hours per day are worked. Some companies allow "pairing" for a position, where two people actually divide work hours of a particular job. Others take increasingly long vacations.

These systems allow the employee to adapt to retirement gradually, and allow for the physical changes and financial adjustments.

Legal Preparation

Prior to retirement, preferably in the thirtieth year of one's life, careful planning with the assistance and advice of a lawyer will do much to avoid problems in the later years of life. For a number of reasons, few Americans do this, and later the lack of a proper will, trouble with landlords, and lack of knowledge about benefits all become sources of worry, particularly after retirement.

Recent legislation makes legal help available, although all of the services planned are not yet fully functional. Lawyers and para-legal personnel are available to all citizens over age 60, regardless of income levels, to assist with wills, estate planning, explanation of government programs, benefits, and rights. The resource persons will be located in senior clubs, at nutrition sites, and other locations on a day-to-day basis. The home state's Bureau of Aging can direct one to these services.

Worries about legal matters and finances are one of the principal concerns of elderly adults, regardless of their financial means. Sound advice from a person they can trust about legal matters can help dispel suspicion and depression. In the past, the cost of these services and lack of knowledge about who to contact has been a deterrent to many persons in need of assistance. These programs should also reduce the amount of fraud aimed at the elderly adult.

DEATH AND DYING

Caring for and assisting a patient who has completed his life's cycle and is near death is one of the most difficult of nursing's functions. It is also a rare privilege to share one's strength in the final hours with another human. This final sharing can give personal satisfaction, or it can be a traumatic experience.

To be of help to the dying patient and his family, the nurse must maintain her own composure. This can only be possible if the nurse has faced and worked through the denial and fears of her own mortality. Although this process is probably never complete in the healthy, active person, one should at least be fairly comfortable with the inevitability of one's own death.

Mourning in our society is almost forbidden. The griever is expected to be brave and to curtail any demonstration of his feelings. This stoic behavior seems to be expected of the elderly patient also. Personnel try to "cheer him up" and seem to set time limits on depression, crying, or other sad behavior. Recovery from the death of a loved one can probably be accomplished less painfully and more quickly if the patient is allowed, or even encouraged, to cry about the loss. Talking about the person and reliving by reminiscence their life-shared experiences may need to be repeated numerous times to facilitate grieving.

Perhaps the process is prolonged for those in nursing homes because they seldom attend the actual funeral, assist in the preparations, or see the deceased after death. Friends and relatives usually attempt to shield them from these experiences. This may be a good method in individual instances, but it deprives the person of facing the reality of death.

To the institutionalized person, other normal methods by which grief is handled are missing. The need to work through the grief by such activities as routine tasks, social relationships, and support of loved ones is reduced in this setting, and the feeling of loss and abandonment seems intensified.

The feelings of helplessness that are experienced by the nurse under these circumstances may lead to avoidance of the patient. A definite nursing plan should be formulated to assist the patient. At least one frequent care giver should be provided to support the patient while he is working through the grief process. The nurse should accept the patient's grieving—which may be expressed by anger, denial, weeping, or general disinterest in life—and express empathy and understanding. Opportunities should be provided over a period of time for the griever to freely express his feelings while the nurse offers feedback on his feelings and supports his value as an individual.

The opportunity for religious guidance and counseling should be offered or provided, when this is the patient's desire. Assuring privacy for minister's visits is essential to good patient care.

Nurses tend to underestimate the time necessary for grief-work to be accomplished by patients, perhaps because their own lives are so dynamic by contrast. The loss of the last relative or friend that a person has from a life of shared experiences must be devastating and is probably mixed with grieving for one's own eventual death. Each individual must face these losses in his own way.

Understanding the Dying Patient

Many of us manage our lives as if we will all be informed of our impending death. A common remark is, "Well, before I die, I will or I want to . . . ," with a variety of activities and desires described. Death comes in many ways. Some are totally unexpected, regardless of age. Some deaths are timed inappropriately, that is, they occur either earlier or later than expected or recovery may take place unexpectedly.

In the past ten years, a great deal has been written about death and dying. Elizabeth Kubler-Ross and others have found that many patients who have not been advised by physician or family of their impending deaths already know this. It is the right of every seriously ill patient to know his diagnosis and that he is near death; and it is the obligation of the physician to so inform the patient. If this obligation is not met by the physician, then it should be met by the registered nurse or other caretakers. The obligation, of course, is only binding when the patient indicates he wishes to know his chances or gives a clear message that he needs answers. The fact that the patient asks probably indicates that he knows and is looking for confirmation. Many patients know they are dying but do not wish to talk about it. Many have spent a lifetime maintaining a calm, serene outlook on life, and to discuss impending death may shatter this calm. Such behavior is unacceptable for them, and only time will enable them to decide on their own method of communication about their dying.

Kubler-Ross and others have indicated the stages through which the dying person usually passes, that is: (1) denial; (2) anger; (3) bargaining; (4) depression; and (5) acceptance. Not all patients have all of these reactions, nor do they occur in this precise order.

It seems logical that by the time in life that admittance to a long-term care facility occurs, the elderly adult has already faced the knowledge of impending death. To many, admittance is synonymous with death. This does not indicate that acceptance of death has been reached, although it may be true in individual instances.

Anger and depression are always present in some elderly patients. Their true source is not always known, although the realization of impending death may be one factor.

Bargaining is common. "If I can only make it until Christmas. . . . I'm going to my daughter's for the holidays. . . . Only six months until I'm 95." Bargaining is a kind of goal setting, and the patient seems at times to miraculously improve and meet the stated objective.

Caring for the Dying Person

How can the nurse learn to care for the dying patient? This care will never be easy. Each person dies as he has lived, in a uniquely individual way, and there are no standard rules to follow. The nurse can begin by attempting to understand her own feelings about the dying patient and to plan how she would want a member of her own family cared for.

One particular area of concern expressed by many students in the care of the dying were the attempts made in hospitals and long-term care facilities to hide the fact that a patient was dying. One of the first things that took place when a patient became critically ill was moving them to a private room near the nursing station. For many patients and visitors, and the dying person, this was a sure sign of approaching death. An attempt to keep a closer watch on the patient (ironical at this time), to save nursing time, and to isolate the terminally ill from others, benefited everyone but the dying person. Isolating him from other people and activities was like pronouncing him dead before his time. Death is a normal part of life, and should be accepted as such, rather than treated as an occurrence to be whispered about and hidden.

If the dying person is not hidden away, particularly in a nursing home, other patients can see him and visit. They can observe the care he receives. The concern of the nursing personnel will assure them that the patient is not abandoned. This helps them be less fearful of their own demise, and the patient benefits from their compassion and by the stimuli of the activity.

Louella Jones had been a resident of Whispering Pines Nursing Home for five years—and had been a favorite of many. She had always helped others and greeted newcomers. As she approached her death, the entire patient group was told she was very ill and that they could visit a few at a time. Some patients read to her, some only patted her hand, some knelt in prayer. Her smile indicated her peace as she told each goodbye. Before her death, while still conscious, she shared with a nurse the joy she felt in being surrounded by her dear friends.

Later, patients related to nurses that they didn't grieve as much as they had felt they would, because they had helped Louella when she needed them. This first experience led to a loose agreement among patients that this type of assistance and involvement should continue and should be extended to assist the family in any way possible. Despite the fact they were dealing with death, morale was enhanced because these patients felt that they were useful and that their services were appreciated by the dying person and by staff personnel.

Moving the patient from his accustomed room seems to be a poor decision, in most instances. The burden this places on a roommate is great, and for his sake, either one or the other probably should be moved, unless there is mutual agreement to remain. Regardless of whether or not the patient is moved, he should be confident that he will not be left alone when he is dying. His door should not be closed, nor curtains drawn. He should not be shut off from his surroundings.

In caring for the terminal patient, communication must be kept open as long as it is possible for the patient to speak. After that—knowing that hearing is the last sense to be lost, the nurse can continue to explain what she is doing. Gentle touch can also be used to express the human concern that is felt for the patient.

During this time the patient may inquire, "Am I worse?" "Am I dying?" or "I'm slipping, aren't I?" The temptation to reassure by saying "Oh, now, you'll be better" must be overcome: to retain the trust of the patient, false reassurances must not be used. But neither should blunt statements be made acknowledging the impending death. Usually rephrasing the question to "Do you feel worse?" or "Why do you feel you're slipping?" will enable the patient to discuss his feelings and thoughts, which is what he desires. The dying person needs help to accept his death, and complete honesty is necessary so that he does not expect the impossible.

No clear set of procedures can be developed for the nurse's behavior as she cares for the dying person. Each patient and circumstance is different, as is each nurse. One nurse may be a skillful physical-care provider, but unable to be effective in supporting the patient and family during the final days. Others can furnish their strength and love to assist the dying. In order to continue to share in stressful situations, nurses must have a method by which their needs are fulfilled.

Physical Care

Of prime importance in the care of the dying is the alleviation of pain. Most people wish to remain in control of themselves and to die with dignity. Pain defeats such a desire. The fear of pain and of losing control is a great part of the fear of death.

The pain medication ordered by the physician should be used generously. If the medication is used routinely, rather than after severe pain is present, it will be more effective. Most persons prefer to remain conscious, to be able to see their families, touch their hands, or to see what goes on around them. Many medications make this impossible. Discussions with the physician may make a change possible, and medications such as those described in hospice care may be substituted. Many people, of course, do not require pain medications, but sometimes a small dosage of a tranquilizer will help them maintain better control.

During the terminal period, the patient should be kept ambulatory for as long as possible. It seems that the human instinct is to put them to bed "to rest." However, as discussed earlier, the dangers of hypomobility only add to the patient's discomfort. Wearing normal daytime apparel will boost morale and help the patient feel a part of normal life.

Many dying persons are bedridden because of severely debilitating diseases. Their care is the same as for any critically ill person. Personal and oral hygiene are extremely important, not only to the patient, but to the family. The physical appearance of the loved one is a comfort to them if they feel and see that the person is well cared for.

As the end of life approaches, decisions must be made about the importance of routinely moving the patient, repositioning, changing dressings, and other procedures that cause pain, anxiety, and are extremely tiring. The patient, if possible, should be making his own decisions about his care. The practical nurse should confer with the registered nurse, the family, and in some instances the physician, in making decisions about discontinuing certain nursing actions. In some instances, the care provided meets the needs of the nurse and/or family, rather than those of the patient.

Reporting Death

In a long-term care facility, a physician is rarely present when a patient dies. A physician must pronounce the patient dead and report the death to the local health department.

When it appears that the patient has died, the nurse attempts to find a pulse, blood pressure, and any respiratory activity. Respiratory activity may be tested by holding a small hand mirror to the nose or mouth and observing it for misting, which would normally occur from the moisture in the breath. She tests for reaction to painful stimuli and pupil response to light. If these are negative, the physician is notified. If the family was not present, the physician notifies the relatives that the death has occurred. The undertaker is then notified, and he takes the patient's body to the nearest hospital where a doctor is available. This physician pronounces the patient dead, and the undertaker transports the body to his establishment. Methods vary in every state for pronouncing death, and facility policies should outline the proper procedures.

The nurse reports the circumstances and the time of death on the patient record. She indicates that the physician was notified, whether or not there were family present, or how they were notified, and which undertaker was summoned. A list of belongings is made, along with a notation as to whether the family removed them or whether they were sent with the body to the mortuary. The undertaker gives a receipt for the possessions if he accepts them, and this is placed with the record.

The care of the body after death depends upon the policies of the institution, which usually accommodate local customs.

REVIEW QUESTIONS

1. What are some of the changes in life style that result from retirement?
2. What methods might be used to make leisure time more useful?
3. Why would it be necessary for the retiree to have supplemental insurance?

4. List at least two ways by which the dying patient can be helped to feel he is not isolated.

5. Explain why some essential nursing care might be discontinued in caring for a dying patient.

6. Why is it good practice to involve relatives in some aspect of terminal care?

BIBLIOGRAPHY

Becker, Ernest. *The Denial of Death.* New York: The Free Press, 1973.

Branter, John. "Positive Approaches to Dying." *Death Education* 1 (1977): 293-304.

Burgess, Karen E. "The Influence of Will on Life and Death." *Nursing Forum* 15 (1976): 239-258.

Dickinson, C. *The Complete Retirement Planning Book.* New York: E.P. Dutton and Company, Inc., 1976.

Dickelman, Nancy. "Pre-Retirement Counseling." *American Journal of Nursing* 78 (August 1978): 1337-1338.

Epstein, Charlotte. *Nursing the Dying Patient.* Reston, Virginia: Reston Publishing Company, 1975.

Fiefel, Herman. *New Meanings of Death.* New York: McGraw-Hill, 1977.

Feinberg, Mortimer et al. *Leavetaking: When and How to Say Goodbye.* New York: Simon & Schuster, 1978.

Fell, James. "Grief Reactions in the Elderly Following Death of a Spouse: The Role of Crises Intervention and Nursing." *Journal of Gerontological Nursing* 3 (November/December 1977): 17-20.

Killian, Bridget Anne. "Attitudes to Death and Bereavement among the Elderly." *World of Irish Nursing* 7 (May 1978): 2-3.

Kubler-Ross, Elizabeth. *Death, the Final Stage of Growth.* N.J.: Prentice-Hall, 1975.

Newman, Joseph, ed. *Plan Your Retirement Now so You Won't Be Sorry Later.* Washington: U.S. News and World Report, Inc. 1974.

Quint, Jeanne C. *The Nurse and the Dying Patient.* New York: Macmillan 1967.

Simms, Lillian. "Dignified Death: A Right, not a Privilege," *Journal of Gerontological Nursing* 1 (November/December 1975): 21-25.

Smith, Cheryl, Sandra Radford et al. "Witnessing Death as Nurses." *Australian Nurses' Journal* 7 (October 1977): 25-27.

chapter 6

The Physical Needs of the Elderly Adult

OBJECTIVES

After studying this unit, the student will be able to:

1. List three dangers of hypomobility and one or more nursing measures to prevent these dangers.

2. Explain why restorative measures planned for the patient may not be successful.

3. Describe the methods for oral care of the unconscious patient, the edentulous patient, and the patient unable to take care of his own oral hygiene.

4. List three causes of pressure sores and several measures to prevent their formation.

5. List three nursing approaches, other than toileting, to be used for a newly admitted patient with urinary incontinence.

6. Describe what benefits can result from the elderly being well groomed.

103

THE RESULTS OF HYPOMOBILITY

The dangers of hypomobility have been the subject of increasing study and research during the past fifteen years, as we have experienced increasing numbers of long-term care facilities throughout the United States and have gained more experience in the care of the elderly adult.

It has been found that reduced activity results in circulatory, metabolic, respiratory, and elimination disturbances. Hypomobility may be voluntary or it may be involuntary. When a spinal cord injury, cerebral vascular accident, or other trauma has occurred, loss of activity is immediate.

Muscular and Bony Changes

Muscular wasting or atrophy occurs when the muscle has experienced loss of nerve impulses; the wasting and weakness cannot be reversed, regardless of exercise. Muscular wasting occurs also when the muscle is not used regularly; strength also diminishes with the wasting. This trend can be reversed with regular exercise, and strength will be improved.

Muscular atrophy occurs rapidly, particulary in the elderly, whose ability to regenerate new cells has slowed. Recovery time is also longer because regeneration is slower. To remain healthy, the bones must experience weight bearing and the tension of muscle contraction and relaxation. As the muscles atrophy, the bones also change, and osteoporosis results. Osteoporotic bones cause pain, are prone to fracture, and the calcium released into the circulatory system may lead to kidney and bladder stones. With disuse, the soft tissues contract, pulling the limbs out of alignment into contractures, limiting the normal range of motion.

Contractures

Contractures occur most frequently in the hip, knee, and shoulder. If a patient spends long periods of time in a chair, or in Fowler's position in bed, knee contractures may result. Pillows under the knee, trochanter rolls, or elevated knee Gatches should never be used, as they impede circulation and cause muscles to contract. Hip flexion contractures occur from soft, saggy mattresses and are most common after hip fractures. Hip flexion can be combatted by using bed boards to provide a firm, straight support to the body. Trochanter rolls placed tightly against the outer thigh, just below the crest of the ilium, will maintain the leg in good position. This position will prevent contractures and outward leg rotation. Many contractures occur after injury or with arthritis when a constant position is maintained to prevent pain to a part.

When I first saw Jenny, she was 34 years old. She was doubled up in a fetal position, her lower limbs so contracted that her thighs were only inches from her chest. Bathing and feeding were difficult. A catheter was necessary because she could not

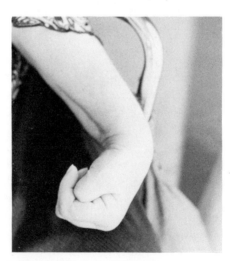

Photographer: Doris Wilson, RN

Contractures must be prevented, they reduce independence and cannot be reversed.

urinate without soiling herself and the bed, regardless of the method used. Her appearance was not very human, although she was bright and uncomplaining. "Mother took very good care of me ever since I got arthritis, but she died last month." The legacy of "care" that refused to cause her daughter pain resulted in an almost completely immobile body and a long life of institutional care.

When patients are unable to move themselves, a footboard is used, with the feet positioned against it at right angles to the legs. If the feet are not supported where muscles are weak, the anterior foot muscles stretch, while the posterior tendon shrinks or contracts, causing foot drop. Only surgery can reverse this deformity, and results are not always successful. If pressing exercises are taught and performed with the feet against the board, circulation is enhanced and muscles may be strengthened.

An alternative method of prevention is the use of plain tennis shoes, with the toes removed so that movement is easy and circulation is not impaired. A recent adaptation of this method, the Space Boot, which is made of plastic and lined with foam, is also useful in prevention of foot drop. This method can be used if the attending physician does not want footboards used. Some authorities believe that footboards do not prevent foot drop, but may be a partial cause of the problem.

In working with these patients, the nurse must acknowledge their discomfort, but must consistently provide positional change, exercise, and positioning to maintain anatomical alignment. Neglecting these activities to avoid the patient's possible complaints or pain is not helpful to the patient, nor does it qualify as good nursing care.

Circulatory Changes

Hypomobility also causes complications in the circulatory system. When circulation slows, there is a stasis of blood in the vessels, and both phlebothrombosis (development of venous thrombi with no inflammation of the vessel) and thrombophlebitis (inflammation of a vein with thrombus formation) may occur in the lower limbs. Both conditions can cause sudden death if the embolus (blood clot) moves and lodges in the lung, causing death to the tissue (pulmonary infarction).

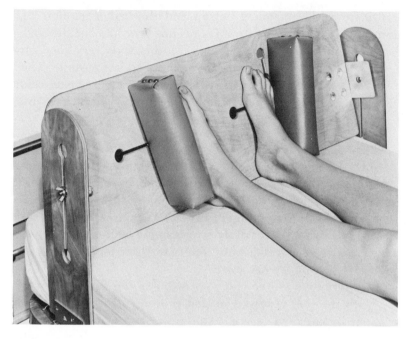

Courtesy F. T. Posey Co.

Footboards prevent slipping down in bed and may prevent foot drop.

Edema of the legs, sacrum, and sacroiliac areas result in circulatory stasis. This lack of circulation to the bony areas makes pressure sores possible and inhibits healing if they are present.

Deterioration of cardiovascular performance also takes place during bedrest. Painful congestion of blood in the feet and legs, vertigo, and fainting are common when a patient assumes an upright position after only a few days of bedrest. When the upright position is assumed, a drop in blood pressure (orthostatic hypotension), palmar sweating, and pallor may occur.

Respiratory Problems of Hypomobility

The inactive or bedfast elderly adult undergoes respiratory changes because of his reduced lung expansion. He does not breathe deeply, and the exchange of oxygen and carbon dioxide is greatly reduced. Mucus secretions are difficult to remove by coughing and become thick and tenacious. These secretions clog the alveoli, and respiratory efficiency is greatly reduced. The patients develop respiratory infections very quickly, as retained secretions are excellent media for bacterial growth, and pneumonia is common in the elderly immobile patient.

A scheduled routine of frequent turning or positional change, whether the patient is in a sitting or lying position, is imperative for the bed patient. If the patient is unable to move, the nurse must reposition him on schedule. Patients should also be instructed to breathe deeply and to cough up secretions. This requires consistent monitoring by the nurse to see that the patient understands and remembers to do so. The patient may be unable to cough up secretions, and other methods of assistance may be necessary. Postural drainage, as described in numerous nursing texts, is also beneficial, although not all elderly adults can tolerate this well. Secretions can be kept liquified by the use of specific drugs and adequate hydration. Medication can also dilate the bronchi and will increase the

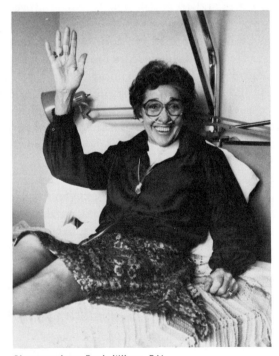

Photographer: Doris Wilson, RN
Model: Iris McKenzie

This patient with respiratory problems remains active and alert.

release of mucus. These methods are more effective when they are used with postural drainage.

The use of intermittent positive-pressure breathing machines such as the Bird or Bennett therapy units may also be beneficial in expanding the lungs and, with the use of nebulized medications, help break up mucus deposits. These machines may be operated by inhalation therapy technicians and by registered or practical nurses. Regardless of who gives the treatment, the nurse is responsible for assisting the patient to cough effectively following the treatment.

If postural drainage is used, cupping and vibration therapy can also be done during the drainage. Cupping is accomplished by holding the hands in a cupped position that traps air between the nurse's hand and the patient's thoracic area. Rhythmic impact is increased with tolerance over the entire area except in the breast area. Vibration is done by placing one hand over the other at an angle, fingers held together, and shaking from the shoulder as if having a chill. This action follows cupping. The patient is then instructed to breathe deeply several times and to cough deeply two or three times. These actions loosen the mucus deposits so they are easier to cough up. The cupping and vibration can also be done without postural drainage, but that is less effective. Extreme care must be taken that the elderly adult is not overfatigued by these methods.

Nurses should take every opportunity to increase the patients' independence, as each task that they do for themselves results in normal respiratory function. Vital signs of the inactive patient should be taken frequently, and observations for cyanosis and dyspnea should be an ongoing routine nursing measure.

Unexpected mental confusion and disorientation of the elderly are frequently the result of inadequate oxygen exchange and developing infections. The use of sedatives may further complicate matters, as deep sleep further depresses both movement and the respiratory system. The patient is best served by vigorous efforts to keep him active and promote movement.

RETENTION OF FUNCTION AND REHABILITATIVE MEASURES

Range-of-motion exercises done routinely during bathing will allow the nurse to identify limitations of motion that need special attention in the patient's daily care. A contracted limb should never be forced through normal range, as such motion is impossible even under anesthesia. If the patient can be tub bathed, some additional range of motion may be possible, as the buoyancy provided by the water lessens the drag of gravity, making movement easier and less painful. Ideally, the patient should be taught the importance of exercises and should be supervised until it can be ascertained that he is doing them correctly. Constant encouragement and praise are needed when the patient assumes this responsibility. A bedside chart that the patient can keep will improve his motivation if the nurse checks it and praises his progress.

If the patient is bedfast, the periodic use of a tilt table (a table that can be tilted from horizontal to vertical by degrees) will aid in assisting the circulatory system to function without stasis of blood. If the patient is being prepared to become ambulatory again, the tilt table can be used to help him adjust to degrees of posture change. Isometric exercises, range of motion exercises, sitting up gradually, and dangling the legs over the edge of the bed before standing are also recommended. These preparations will help prevent orthostatic hypotension and vertigo as blood is drained from the upper body to

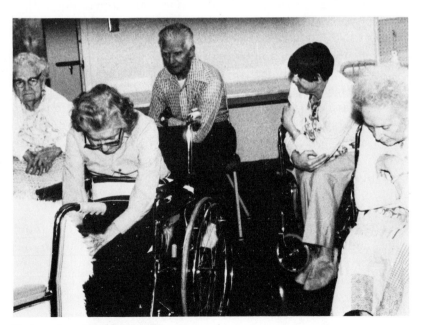

Photographer: Doris Wilson, RN
Models: Marian B. Murphy, Clarence Bloyd, Beulah Kay, Alice E. Hallmark

An exercise class works to maintain muscular function.

the lower. Gradual weight bearing is also accomplished by this method after a long period of hypomobility.

To summarize, the nurse's responsibilities for rehabilitation of patients include the following:

1. Planning, executing or directing, and evaluating frequent changes of position, according to individual needs.
2. Either doing for or teaching the patient bed exercises. These may be range of motion, leg raising and flexing, situps, or pulling up on trapezes.
3. Arranging beds, bedside tables, and overbed tables for the patient's convenience so that he is as self-sufficient as possible.
4. Planning with the patient for a bowel and bladder retraining program.
5. Teaching the patient to feed, dress, and toilet himself using any devices adapted for such measures.
6. Teaching and evaluation of the use of canes, crutches, wheelchairs, or other prosthetic devices, in cooperation with the physical therapist.

When the patient's need for rehabilitative treatment is beyond the expertise of the nurse, the doctor will write specific orders for restorative treatment by the physical therapist. The nurse's responsibility is to assure continuity of care, following the directions of the physical therapist, which have been demonstrated and have been noted on the patient's care plan. The therapist will spend a given amount of time with the patient, usually on a five-day schedule. To ensure progress by the patient, the treatment must be taken over by nursing personnel in the interim between the therapist's visits and repeated frequently during the day.

The need for other rehabilitative services as a result of trauma, stroke, and other chronic diseases may be present. The physician may order that these services be provided by other health disciplines, such as occupational therapy, speech therapy, and social services. To have these services available, the patient would need to be in a skilled care facility. In some instances, because one or more of these services were not furnished locally, the patient would need to be transferred to where the services were available. This may not be economically or logistically practical.

Mental problems as a result of inactivity have been discussed in Chapter 3. Confusion and disorientation can occur within a few days, so precarious is the balance of some elderly persons' mental health. Activity and stimulus are essential to their mental health, as well as their physical well-being.

Attitudes Concerning Rehabilitative Measures

In many long-term care facilities, rehabilitation is mostly lip service; the goals stated on patient care plans are rarely accomplished. A room set aside for physical therapy may be unused, with staff persons unaware of the uses for some of the expensive equipment stored there. Many feel that restoration of function in the aged is impossible and is a waste of time. This attitude is easily relayed to patients and families, as it is from one nurse to another. The health professions

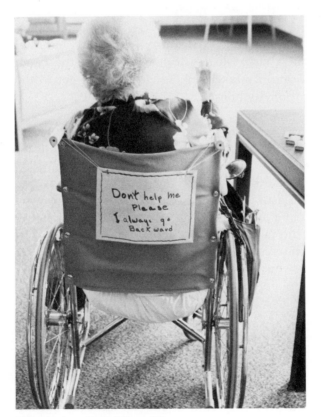

Photographer: Doris Wilson, RN

Independence must be encouraged and respected.

have not always assumed the leadership that is necessary to ensure effective geriatric rehabilitation.

Regardless of the availability and use of excellent rehabilitative measures, not all elderly people (nor younger ones) benefit from efforts to improve physical function. Much of the success of a program depends upon the patient himself. If he has a goal and some supportive family or friends, the program is much more likely to succeed than if he is alone in the world, feels defeated, and has a poor self-image.

Although the average long-term care facility is not a sophisticated rehabilitation center, it should strive to promote independence. Nurses should assess patients for what they can do, rather than for their failings. Success must be counted in small improvements that can be realistically accomplished, rather than startling revisions.

> Mrs. Burton, who needed to be fed every morsel, with firm encouragement and support, can now handle her toast and other finger foods. Fred Murry, who is almost blind and used to sit in a chair all day, can now follow the handrails to the identification marker on the elevator and get to the first-floor dining room by himself.

These changes may seem too insignificant to be noted, but they greatly improved the quality of life for these patients and increased their self-esteem.

If the nurse has a positive attitude ("I know it can be done") and is enthusiastic about assisting the elderly, progress is possible. Family must be involved in this exciting challenge, and every person working in the facility must be interested enough to reward the patient by his interest, concern, and active friendliness.

Patients must not be allowed to sit and regress. They must be stimulated and urged to move, achieve, and change.

> A 16-year-old high-school student, employed for the summer in a nursing home, was observed singing and holding Josh Remke, her 85-year-old patient, in a dancing position. She didn't know that the hesitant, shuffling steps he was taking were his first since admission a month ago. Professional measures had proven worthless, and he had been shelved as "hopeless." As Rose continued to coax, sing, and "bully" him that

summer, he became fully independent in activities of daily living and became able to walk the length of the hall several times a day. Unorthodox methods were used, but simple concern and unawareness of the cultural and professional expectations formulated by nursing staff and physicians for this elderly man resulted in tremendous gains for a man who had sat down to die.

GENERAL NURSING MEASURES FOR THE ELDERLY

The Pressure Sore

One of the dangers of inactivity is the decubitus ulcer or pressure sore. To many lay and professional people, the "bed sore" is synonymous with the nursing home.

It is estimated that treating a decubitus ulcer costs from $5,000 to $7,000. The pain, both physical and mental, to the patient cannot be estimated. Pressure sores may require surgical treatment and hospitalization, and may even be a cause of death.

Pressure sores may develop at any bony prominence, such as the sacrum, the shoulder blade, ischial tuberosities, the trochanters, heels, and elbows. Decubiti start as small, reddened areas or indentations in the skin. The area first becomes reddened, in some instances a bleb appears, and the area undergoes darkening. The tissue may become hard, and necrosis of the tissue develops, with sloughing, leaving an ulcer. Without care, this can enlarge to such an extent that the underlying bony structure may be exposed. Infection may occur to further complicate the problem. Body fluid, protein, and electrolytes are lost from the site. With proper care, regeneration can occur within a short time. Healing may take much longer, however, and in some instances, regardless of the care, the decubti only enlarge. Much depends upon the size of the ulcer and the patient's general condition.

Chronic and temporary risks

High-risk patients may be thought of in two cateogories, either chronic or temporary. Chronic risks are those patients—young old— with loss of mobility, such as cord injuries, cerebral vascular accidents, multiple sclerosis, terminal carcinoma, Parkinson's disease, organic brain syndrome, chronic alcoholism, or severe arthritis.

Those patients who are temporary risks are those in casts, drug addicts, and those needing narcotics. Any patient considered cachectic has lost muscle and fat padding from his bony frame and has no cushion against any type of pressure. His risk is usually both temporary and high.

Causes of pressure sores

Any patient who has a poor nutritional level, particularly a diet deficient in sufficient protein and vitamin content, or any problems of adsorption of nutrients and a low hemoglobin, is prone to skin problems.

Pressure, which deprives the tissue of oxygen and nutrients, or an injury to the skin such as a bruise, pinching of a cast, or abrasion of delicate tissue on rough wadded bedding may cause decubiti.

Any skin problems will be complicated if the tissue is wet from urine, feces, or perspiration. Edematous tissue is also more prone to breakdown than is normal tissue. Prolonged contact with urine alone may cause maceration and skin breakdown.

Prevention of pressure sores

If proper assessment is done upon admission and observations are made daily with a good light, the nurse can identify the decubiti-prone patient. Upon admission, when a thorough physical assessment is done, the nurse should observe and describe in her notes any pressure sore present, any break in the skin, or any reddened areas that seem to be potential problems. Problems noted should also be reported to the head nurse. The integrity of the skin is of vital importance in preventing avenues for secondary infections.

Position change

All patients with limited mobility, but particularly high-risk patients, must have vigorous, continuous nursing care. The patient's position must be changed at least every two hours. A schedule posted on the bed or door may help in maintaining the proper rotation of positions throughout the 24 hours. The patient should be propped with pillows to maintain his position; the body should be in anatomical alignment, with no two body surfaces in contact. Sliding down in bed can be corrected by lowering the headrest somewhat. Do not elevate the knee Gatch, or use pillows under the knees, as this promotes venous stasis. Footboards will also assist in preventing the patient from slipping down in bed. Overhead trapeze bars for patients who can use them are helpful to the patient and nurse in moving and also in maintaining muscular strength. Changing the patient's position in bed should always be done with the aid of a lifting sheet, which should extend from the shoulder to beneath the buttocks, to reduce the friction (sheet burns) on fragile skin caused by pulling movements.

Patients who are bedfast are not the only ones in danger of developing decubiti. If the patient is in a wheelchair, without position change regularly, his skin is prone to breakdown. This may be further complicated by incontinency and perspiration. There is a large variety of wheelchair inflatables, flotation pads, multiplastic gels, and other cushions designed to conform to the patient's contours. They are helpful and comfortable, but a definite schedule for changing position is more important. A timer attached to the chair and set for specific intervals will remind the patient to lift himself for a position change. The use of rubber rings or "doughnuts" is prohibited as they interfere with nutrition to that area of skin positioned in the middle of the ring.

Skin care

Elderly patients, whose skin is dried and flaky, should not be bathed every day, nor should soap be used if it can be avoided, as it further dries the skin. If soap is used, it should be rinsed off well and thoroughly dried. Gentle massage over bony areas, or any reddened skin area, should be done at bath times and whenever the patient is turned. The liberal use of bath oils, lotions, softening agents and other skin emollients is highly recommended. Precautions must be taken so that the skin does not become macerated from overuse of these products.

The use of sheepskins (artificial ones that can be laundered) under the buttocks, and heel and elbow guards, is usually helpful. Water beds are ideal for high-risk patients, as are alternating pressure mattresses. If the patient is cared for at home, inexpensive inflatable camping mattresses are useful. If water-filled mattresses are used, adequate precaution should be taken against the use of sharp objects and pins, which might rupture the material. Surgical gloves filled with water and secured tightly can be used for heel and elbow guards to provide further protection from pressure and friction. Commercial gel pads are also available.

The causes of decubiti should be explained to high-risk patients and their families. Family members should be taught which are the danger areas for formation of the sores and encouraged to assist by examination and massage of endangered areas when they visit. Most persons are very receptive and are eager to be able to do something for their family member.

Treatment of pressure sores

There are numerous remedies for healing decubiti. If any medication, salves, or ointments are used, a doctor's order for their use must be obtained. Most long-term care facilities have nursing service policies that cover the treatment of decubiti. If the individual physician does not agree with the policy, he may countermand the order with his own preference. Regardless of what policy is followed, it should be clearly understood by nursing personnel so that time is not lost in beginning treatment and so that care is persistent.

In most instances, the best treatment seems to be the least—to depend on the curative powers of the patient's body. Prevention by constant observation, scheduled movement, and massage of bony areas is far better than any treatment. The patient should be positioned so that pressure is removed from the affected area. The area should be cleansed of all necrotic tissue or other debri. This can be done with mild soap and water, hydrogen peroxide, povidone iodine (Betadine) or other agents, according to policy.

A number of effective debriding solutions are available that will aid in cleaning the sore and may be ordered by the doctor. Skin grafting, which will require hospitalization, may be necessary if there is extensive loss of tissue.

Keeping the wound dry hastens healing, and while many methods are available, a gooseneck lamp with a standard light bulb, placed at least 18 inches from the body, is among the most efficient and safest. It may be necessary to use a heat cradle to help keep the patient warm and shielded for privacy as the wound dries in the air. This exposure to the air will promote exudate drying, which encourages tissue regeneration and protects against infection.

A new method of treatment in which the pressure sore is covered with preparations usually used with stomal care has been reported. The procedure has proved successful in treating pressure sores in different phases of development.

Any patient with a pressure sore should have his temperature checked at least daily. Some elevation is normal as dead cells are adsorbed by the body's circulation. If the temperature is elevated over 101°, or above the patient's normal baseline temperature, the physician should be notified.

The need for positioning the patient so that pressure on the affected area is relieved may call for an abnormal position for the patient. The need for these measures must be constantly emphasized to prevent frustration, hostility, and depression. Additional time should be scheduled for supporting this patient with encouragement and frequent attention. Visitation from other patients should be encouraged, and the activity director should be alerted to plan diversional activities if possible.

In some instances, regardless of intensive preventative measures, skin breakdown does occur. There are many pressure sores that do not respond to treatment. The presence of these sores does not always denote poor care, but may simply reflect the physical health of the patient.

Incontinence

Incontinencies of either urine or stool, or both, are a serious problem in the care of the elderly patient. The American culture puts great emphasis on the early successful toilet training of children. It is one of the first accomplishments that is praised and valued by parents. As an adult, the inability to control body functions results in feelings of guilt, shame, failure, and anticipation of censure by others.

There are several types of urinary dysfunctions. Overflow incontinence is a constant loss of small amounts of urine. Stress incontinence is the intermittent loss of urine when the person is under either physical or mental stress. This occurs frequently in women, particularly when laughing, coughing, or straining, and is not limited to the elderly. Dysfunction may be so severe that there is a complete inability to retain urine.

Incontinence of urine has many causes, such as:

1. Muscular weakness of the pelvic floor in women.
2. The nerve supply to the bladder has been destroyed by spinal or brain injury.

3. Destruction of tissue from irradiation treatment.

4. Infections of the urinary tract.

5. Destruction of the urinary sphincter after surgery or injury.

It also seems that much of the incontinence found in the elderly adult in the nursing home is due not to loss of functional ability, but to neglect. If the patient needs to be assisted to the toilet, or needs a urinal or bedpad and must always wait for help, incontinence of necessity will occur and become a habit. Incontinence may also be a result of isolation and boredom or depression. To the completely dependent patient who is denied normal stimulation, love, acceptance, and evidence of self-worth, this may be the one way he can demonstrate independence and maintain a semblance of control over others. Incontinence gains attention and action if no other method is successful. Incontinence can become a habit, causing voluntary control to be lost. The use of infantilizing measures such as diapers and pads further reduces self-esteem and these methods meet nursing needs rather than patient needs.

Perineal and catheter care

The long-term use of catheters to maintain dryness is not advisable unless there are obstructions that prevent normal urine flow. The incidence of urinary-tract infections with constant use of indwelling catheters is high, and the infection may prove fatal. Urinary infections in the elderly adult are frequently asymptomatic, and the infection may be overwhelming prior to diagnosis and treatment. Indwelling Foley catheters should be used only when the patient is unconscious or there is no hope that urinary continence can be achieved by other methods.

A leg bag can be used as a collection bag for indwelling catheters for both male and female patients. These bags make ambulation easier, as the large collection bag used at the bedside is conspicuous, awkward, and a source of embarrassment. The leg bag should not be used when the patient is in bed, however, as this increases the danger of backflow and infection. If the patient uses a leg bag, he must be instructed in the proper sterile technique to assure the cleanliness of his catheter's connection to the bedside bag. If he is unable to manage, the practical nurse must attend to the connection.

Leg bags must be cleaned each night to prevent odors. A solution of 1 tablespoon of vinegar to 1 quart of water will deodorize. If the male patient has an indwelling catheter for a long period, the end of the catheter should be taped to the abdomen. This prevents inflammation and possible ulceration at the penile-scrotal angle. The glans and the urethra are relieved of pressure from the position of the penis. The drainage tube should be fastened to the bed to prevent the weight of the tubing from pulling the catheter and applying pressure on the urinary meatus and the penis. A rubber band looped around the tube and secured by a safety pin to the bed linen will eliminate pull, and allow the patient to turn freely without putting traction on the catheter.

When indwelling catheters are in use, the perineal area must be kept immaculately clean to prevent infections and to decrease odors. The male patient is usually better cared for in this regard, but the female patient with an indwelling catheter may not have adequate care. The female's labia should be carefully separated and cleansed with soap and water. A separate wash cloth, preferably of the disposable type, should be used for each stroke, the movement always from anterior to posterior. Pouring water over the vulva is an efficient method of rinsing. A clean set of cloths is used for drying.

As the catheter extends from the external urinary meatus, it becomes soiled with natural secretions, perhaps some urinary leakage, or blood. If the catheter is not kept clean, the materials may cause local irritation and odor or cause infection to travel up the urethra. Each time perineal (crotch) care is given, the catheter should be cleansed with benzalkonium (zephrian) chloride, peroxide, Betadine preps, or surgical soap.

Indwelling catheters are always a possible source of infection. An external condom catheter (Texas catheter) can be used to keep the male patient dry. If this method is to be used, the patient must be free from urethral obstructions and infection. The skin of the penis must also be free from any inflammation.

The condom catheter is a latex product and is elastic. Extreme care must be used so that the device does not cause circulatory problems. After the penis has been cleansed with soap and water and dried, the condom, which comes from the manufacturer rolled up, is gently rolled over the penis up to 2 inches behind the head of the penis, leaving approximately ½ inch slack at the connecting end of the catheter. The slack prevents the end of the penis from rubbing against the end of the condom, causing discomfort or irritation. A foam adhesive strip is supplied with the catheter. The adhesive is placed over the top of the condom catheter just below the rolled edge of the condom. It should be snug enough to prevent escape of urine, and as the tape is expandable, there is little danger of constriction. Ordinary tape should not be used. The condom is then connected to a bedside drainage unit or to a leg bag. The top of the drainage tubing should be taped to the inner thigh to prevent pulling on the condom. The condom should be removed each day, and the penis cleansed with mild soap and water and dried thoroughly. A period of air drying will also prevent skin breakdown. The condom should be replaced every second day.

There are a number of widely used standardized programs to achieve urinary and fecal continence. Each facility should have these procedures or similar ones available, and personnel should understand how they work and the importance of continuity in their use.

The nurses' attitude about retraining programs is felt by the patient and has a decided effect upon their success. A calm, positive approach inspires hope in the patient and family. The patient should never be treated as a child, and the problems of incontinence should be thoroughly discussed. Plans for reversing the problem and the methods to be used are made with the patient. The following measures may be of help in ensuring the success of the retraining program.

1. Keep the patient out of bed if at all possible.
2. Insist that the patient wear street clothes and attend to grooming details.
3. During the retraining period, keep the patient socially acceptable, using the uro-sheath for males and protective underwear for females, to prevent embarrassment if an accident occurs.
4. Take the patient to the bathroom or use bedside commodes, not bedpans or urinals.
5. Get him involved in activities; keep him stimulated.
6. Be sure he has an adequate fluid and roughage intake.
7. Use touch generously.

Urinary and rectal incontinence may take months to reverse. Success may not be complete. It is, however, a positive step, one that says, "We care, you are valued, we can succeed."

ORAL HEALTH CARE

In institutions where the residents are all elderly, and the majority may be endentulous, the oral care of the patient may be neglected.

When the patient is admitted, nursing personnel should examine the mouth as they make their assessment of the patient. Some pertinent points to cover are as follows:

1. How many of his own teeth does the patient have? What is their general condition?
2. If he does not have teeth, does he have dentures? Are they in good repair? Do they fit properly?
3. Can he do his own oral hygiene?
4. Does the gingival mucosa have any ulcers, lesions? Are the gums healthy (light pink)?
5. Does the patient report he is able to chew his food properly?

The condition of the mouth and teeth should be reported to the physician if any abnormalities are found. Any dental problem can adversely affect the patient's general health. His general health will also affect his mouth, gums, and teeth.

Many of the present elderly population never learned proper oral care. Instruction can be done in groups, but preferably individual follow-up must be done. Some important points to remember in teaching proper care are:

1. The brush should be small and soft, with a small number of bristles, so it can reach all of the teeth effectively.
2. The grooves and biting surfaces as well as the area between gums and teeth need to be brushed to remove bacteria and waste.
3. To clean between gums and teeth, the brush is angled at 45°.
4. The use of a brush in this fashion may result in some bleeding from the gums, but this will cease in a few days.
5. The gums should be gently massaged with the finger.

If the patient has hemophilia or leukemia or any symptoms of mouth bleeding, or is taking anticoagulant drugs (heparin) or chemotherapeutic agents such as methotrexate, which may cause mouth ulcers, the use of a toothbrush is contraindicated: gauze squares, terry face-cloths, or cotton swabs should be used for cleaning with frequent medicated mouth rinses.

Dentifrices are not necessary in oral hygiene, but if they are used, they should not be strong enough to harm soft tissue. The American Dental Association seal of approval on the container is a reliable mark of safety. The teeth should be flossed daily, with flat, unwaxed dental floss. Realistically, it will be impossible for all patients to do this because of arthritic changes in their hands. Others, not accustomed to routine tooth care will not form this habit. The nurse's responsibility is to see that floss, brushes, and dentrifice are available for those able to use them. She should remind patients to do oral hygiene, and check for compliance, but not belabor the point.

For those patients with dentures, a brush, cleaning agents, and a safe dental cup for overnight storage are necessary. If the patient is unable to clean his dentures, the nurse should clean them. Many persons feel self-conscious about their need for dentures, so the nurse should do this care as unobtrusively as possible. Patients usually have a special powder for cleaning the dentures, but soap or any dental powder is permissible. The use of running water rather than a basin makes the job easier. A wash cloth placed in the basin will prevent breakage of the plates if they are accidentally dropped. Hot water should never be used, as the materials from which plates are made are distorted by heat. Some of the materials used in the manufacture of plates also absorb food, and plates become odoriferous unless well cleaned. Commercial immersion cleaners are recommended for this purpose, although efficient ones can be made. The commercial types contain chemicals that can be harmful if swallowed, but a solution of one tablespoon of vinegar in 8 ounces of water is a safe and effective substitute to use with the elderly, who may become confused.

The patient who wears dentures should be encouraged to wear them throughout the day. If he does not, prompt investigation as to the causes should be made. In many instances, it may be because the dentures are ill-fitting or loose. Poorly fitted dentures can traumatize the soft tissues of the mouth. Powders and lining materials may help in some cases of problems with loose plates. If new dentures are needed, or if professional assistance is needed to adjust the fit, the problem may be more difficult.

The Unconscious Patient

When the patient is unable to care for himself or is comatose, the mouth must be cared for by the nurse. If the patient is helpless or vomiting, or unconscious, dentures should be removed, as they may obstruct the airway. Otherwise, routine care should be done. In addition, the gums should be gently massaged and the tongue cleaned. The use of cotton-tipped swabs is contraindicated, as the cotton will not pick up mucus deposits: gauze pads, or terry facecloths wrapped around the nurse's gloved finger are more effective. Care should be taken not to cause a gag reflex, nor to use liquids that may cause choking or aspiration.

If the patient has teeth, a toothbrush should not be used, unless it is used dry to prevent aspiration. A terry facecloth covering the finger may be rubbed across the teeth. A padded tongue blade placed between the teeth may need to be used in all of these procedures to prevent the patient from biting down on the nurse's fingers.

The lips and oral mucosa should be kept moist, as the unconscious person usually breathes through the mouth and is not taking liquids or foods that promote the formation of saliva. The most commonly used preparation is glycerin and lemon juice swabs. Petroleum jelly or lanolin can be used on the lips. Oral care should be performed frequently for the unconscious, at least three times daily, or more often if the patient is running a temperature.

The Dental Consultant

Each skilled-level nursing home must have a consultant dentist. This person should be one interested in prevention of dental problems and in teaching. In-service programs to teach nursing personnel proper methods of oral care may be part of the dentist's contribution to patient care. A dental hygienist can also play an important part in the oral care of patients if the institution is fortunate enough to have the services of one.

The dental consultant assures the facility that dental care for patients will be available if the patient has no private dentist. If a patient must visit the dentist for the removal of a tooth, replacement should be made, as the loss of teeth causes nutritional, digestive, and eventually jaw alignment problems. With the present system of financing care for the elderly, this may prove impossible unless the patient or family can pay for the care themselves. Some county governments may furnish this service, and some service clubs contribute monies for such emergencies.

PERSONAL GROOMING

The American public spends millions of dollars each year on grooming aids. Our media bombard us on the appropriate cosmetic for retaining our youth and beauty. We all become appearance conscious at an early age. The industry is not interested in reaching the elderly, who have the greatest need, it would seem, for their products. Nursing personnel also seem to assume at times that appearance is not important to the elderly adult except for cleanliness. The morale boost that results in knowing that you are well groomed is widely understood, but the principle is not always well applied by health-care workers.

What kind of grooming problems are common in the elderly? As the male ages, in many instances he loses some or all of his scalp hair. His beard becomes thinner, but body hair remains much the same. Unfortunately, as the desirable hair is lost, the eyebrows may grow quite bushy, and nasal and ear hair also grows. Body hair on the female tends to decrease, and the scalp hair may also become very thin. Facial hair, on the upper lip and chin, may begin to grow quite profusely. Our culture values attractive hair, but does not condone excess body hair. Facial hair on the female is particularly at variance with our ideals, and very upsetting to the woman.

These changes bother people to different degrees, but they nearly always distress, and may even make the patient repugnant to family and friends. To retain a comfortable self-image, most people would like superflous hair removed. The hair can be safely removed by tweezer, by shaving, by cutting with a scissors, or by depilatories or wax applications, according to its location. Hair in the ears and nose can be removed by clipping with small scissors or tweezers. Shaving is probably the easiest method for removal of facial hair. Contrary to popular belief, shaving does not hasten the growth of facial hair. Shaving is also easier than the use of a depilatory, which may cause skin irritations, and is rather costly.

In many instances, women seem to fare better than men in receiving nursing assistance with grooming. This is probably related to

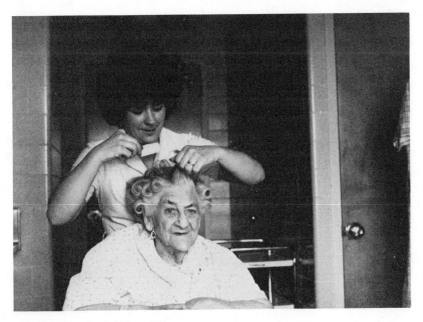

Photographer: Doris Wilson, RN
Models: Agnes Cox (patient), Linda Stanley

A new hairdo and earrings boost morale.

the fact that most nurses are females, and are better acquainted with the woman's needs. It must be accepted that being well shaved is as important to the male's feeling of well-being as is any grooming measure for the female.

Shampooing the hair for bed patients or ambulatory patients should be as routine as bathing. Hairdryers are of great assistance in hastening the drying of the hair.

Care of fingernails, especially for the bedfast, is most important. Confused patients may scratch themselves and, particularly if the nails are dirty, can cause infections. Cleaning and cutting the fingernails should become part of the bath care of patients. Nails should never be cut shorter than below the point where the nails emerge from the skin. If the person is ambulatory, he still may need help with nail care. Volunteers or family members might be asked to assist with this aspect of patient care.

The care of the toenails of the elderly adult is very important. Infections that are frequent with ingrown toenails, improperly cut nails, or skin breaks due to improper use of tools may endanger the life of the patient, particularly the diabetic.

If the patient showers, or is bedfast, the feet should be soaked in warm water and the nails cleaned with a file, which will prevent nail thickening. Gentle friction by use of a wash cloth will assist in removal of dead skin and calluses. Corns or bunions should never be tampered with, but should be called to the attention of the charge nurse and noted on the patient's record. Toenails can be cut straight across when the nail has softened, unless there is infection or redness present, except in the case of the diabetic. A podiatrist usually makes routine calls at the facility and manages the care of the diabetics' feet or other patients who have problems. Daily soaking of nails will keep them soft and manageable.

The practical nurse should be aware of the facility's policies of foot care for the diabetic. Most institutions do not allow nurses' assistants to cut nails, and the LPN must know if she is permitted to do so. Someone other than a podiatrist must be able to cut nails, as they cannot be neglected between visits.

Personal grooming must not be separated from routine nursing care, but rather be an integral part of it. It is an important part of our self-image, which needs to be maintained and enhanced at every opportunity.

REPORTING AND RECORDING

As the practical nurse cares for the patient, or supervises his care, she observes changes in the patient's physical and mental condition and his vital signs. She may be starting new treatments or observing the results in ongoing ones. Some of the data she collects must be reported, either to the physician, the registered nurse, or the supervisor. Some data must be both reported and recorded, some only recorded on the patient's record.

Most nurses dislike entering data on records, perhaps because they are more skillful in oral reporting than in making written comments. The importance of concise notes that portray what is happening to the patient is as important as physical care and is an integral part of nursing, not to be divided from any other care task.

The types of nursing notes used vary from the more traditional narrative type to the problem-oriented type. The nursing notes of the

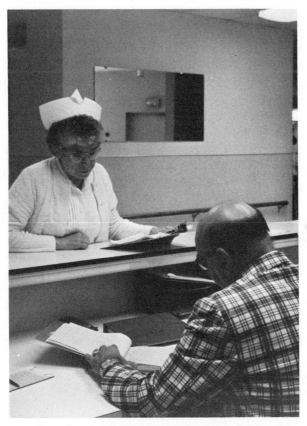

Photographer: Doris Wilson, RN
Models: Jerome M. Hansen, Dolores Byer

The physician reviews the patient's record to assess the patient's progress and as a basis for his orders.

acutely ill person in the hospital vary from those required in a long-term care facility. State and federal regulations have different standards for intermediate and skilled nursing care facilities. The nurse therefore, must be aware of the requirements of the facility in which she is employed. The nursing policy manual should explain specifically the agencies' standards for nursing notes and other patient record entries.

The nurses' notes could be seen as a tool of accountability. Accountability is that obligation to report, explain, and justify nursing actions. Nurses have the obligation to be accountable to their patients, employers, and to each other. The nurses' notes could be visualized as an itemized account of what has been done. If the action has not been charted, there is no proof it has been done, and the nurse has no method of explaining her actions.

The patient's record can be subpoenaed as evidence in court trials. Nurses are customarily warned about the legal implications of their practice, and some chart superfluous information in an attempt to clarify nursing action. This occurs particularly during unusual occurrences, such as patient injuries due to falls or unexpected changes in the patient's condition. If the facility's policy manual is clearly written, and the nurse adheres to the policies, and the notes describe problems from beginning to conclusion, legal requirements will also be satisfied.

State and Medicare surveyors from around the nation who were attending classes sponsored by the Department of Health, Education and Welfare (HEW) reported that the most frequent problem encountered in their evaluations of nurses' notes on the patient record was the lack of continuity in describing what happened to the patient.

> 2/17/79—Patient found on floor of bathroom, states he fell when "leg wobbled." Abrasion and hematoma found on left shoulder, elbow, and hip. No complaint of pain. When lifted by three nurses back to bed, he cried out "My hip, my hip." Dr. J. Doe notified.
>
> 2/18/79—Continues to complain of pain.

The notes continue, but one month later, they have not stated whether the doctor visited, whether X-rays had been taken, or whether the pain was still present. However, if the chart was examined, the physician's order for X-rays was found present. Questioning of the nurses revealed that the patient had been taken by ambulance to a hospital, X-rays were taken, and no fracture was found. If the records had been used in court, none of these facts would have been revealed, and the doctor's orders would appear not to have been carried out. There was no indication that the pain was gone, nor that the abrasions and hematoma had been treated, nor that they healed.

Anything that happens to a patient, or any complaint he makes, must be resolved by carrying through and describing the progression and final outcome on the records. Any treatment must be described, as well as the patient's reaction to it.

2/17/79   Decubitus on outer aspect of left ankle cleaned with normal saline, dried, and heat lamp applied for 10 minutes.

This entry does not tell us of progress in healing, whether the area has enlarged since the last treatment, and whether it is infected, or whether the patient is apprehensive about the treatment or experiences pain. Several days passed with no notation of treatment. Was it done? Was the area healed? These examples show how poor charting does not give a continuous report of the patient's condition and could be interpreted as negligence.

Another method of communication used in nursing is verbal reporting. The nurses's assistant reports to the registered or licensed practical nurse or the practical nurse reports to the registered nurse as a normal chain of command. As the personnel work with patients, changes in the patient's condition, patient's complaints that they are unable to handle, or many other incidents must be related to the nurse in charge. She is responsible for the care of the patients on the unit and must be kept informed.

For communication to occur, there must be a sender and a receiver. If the receiver does not correctly interpret the message, communication has not occurred. The message must be concise and accurate.

The reports of any care giver to the charge nurse, or the report of any student nurse to the licensed staff, must be carefully noted and appropriate follow-up made. The charge nurse is always busy and may be the only licensed personnel on the unit. If she is to depend upon her staff for pertinent information, then she must value their reports and her attention to their observation must be prompt and thorough. If staff communicate and see that nothing is done, their observations seem useless, and communication breaks down.

Inattention to staff observations can have serious repercussions to the patient. Changes in vital signs, state of consciousness, reddened skin areas, disorientation, or other observations must have immediate follow-up. They are symptoms of serious emergency conditions or of problems that must have immediate care to prevent future deterioration.

Most observations by nursing personnel can be given to the charge nurse during a brief report on the condition of patients cared for during the day. Morning reports can clue the caretaker in on anticipated problems of specific patients, but all care givers should be made aware of what is considered a priority report that must be communicated immediately.

REVIEW QUESTIONS

1. What type of muscular wasting can be reversed? Explain how this can be done.
2. Name at least three results other than muscular wasting that occur with hypomobility. How can they be reversed?
3. Where do pressure sores usually occur and what are some of the early symptoms?
4. List at least three causes of decubiti.
5. List at least three important steps in oral care of the unconscious patient.
6. Why is good grooming important to the elderly adult?

RECOMMENDED ACTIVITIES

1. Demonstrate range of motion for a bedrest patient on a fellow student.
2. With another nursing student, practice brushing your partner's teeth. Discuss what bothered you as your teeth were cleaned. How could you eliminate this discomfort?
3. Develop a nursing-care plan for an incontinent patient that includes all aspects of care that would be helpful in reversing incontinence.
4. With a group of classmates, make a list of grooming standards you feel are essential to the elderly adult's self-esteem. Evaluate ten patients and judge whether these patients meet your list of standards.

BIBLIOGRAPHY

Cameron, Gerry. "Pressure Sores: What to Do When Prevention Fails." *Nursing '79* 19 (January, 1979): 43-47.

Campbell, Claire. *Nursing Diagnosis and Intervention in Nursing Practice*. New York: John Wiley & Sons, 1978, pp. 1453, 1593, 1591, 1598, 1601.

Cuica, Rudy et al. "Active Range of Motion Exercises." *Nursing '78* 8 (August 1978): 45–49.

De Christopher, Judith. "Factors Important in Geriatric Rehabilitation: Need Age Be a Liability?" *Association of Rehabilitative Nurses Journal* 2 (July/ August 1977): 9-16.

Frankel, Laurence J., and Betty B. Richard. "Exercises Help the Elderly Live Longer." *Nursing '77* 7 (December 1977): 58-63.

Goldman, Ralph. "Rest; Its Use and Abuse in the Aged." *Journal of the American Geriatrics Society* 25 (October 1977): 433-437.

Henderson, Virginia, and Gladys Nite. *Principles and Practice of Nursing*. New York: Macmillan 1978, pp. 319-375, 1541-1548.

Hirschberg, Gerald. "Promoting Patient Mobility." *Nursing '77* 7 (May 1977): 42-47.

Kavchak-Keys, Mary Anne. "Treating Decubitus Ulcers Using Four Proven Steps." *Nursing '77* 7 (October 1977): 44-45.

_____. "Four Proven Steps for Preventing Decubitus Ulcers." *Nursing '77* 7 (September 1977): 58-61.

Larkin, Patricia D., and Barbara A. Backer. *Problem-Oriented Nursing Assessment*. New York: McGraw-Hill, 1977.

Leinweber, Eileen. "Belts to Make Moves Smoother." *American Journal of Nursing* 78 (December 1978): 2080-2081.

Luckman, Joan, and Karen C. Sorenson. *Medical-Surgical Nursing*. Philadelphia: W. B. Saunders Co., 1974, p. 716-720.

_____. *Perspective: In Working with Older People*. Vol. II: Biological, Psychological and Sociological Aspects of Aging. U.S. Department of Health, Education and Welfare, Public Health Service Publication, 1972.

chapter 7

Safety Measures: Environment and Drugs

OBJECTIVES

After studying this unit, the student will be able to:

1. List four physical problems that may precipitate accidents in the elderly.

2. Describe the precautions necessary in using safety straps or shoulder halters in wheelchairs and beds.

3. List the points necessary in quality charting concerning the use of restraints.

4. Explain four reasons why drugs may react differently than anticipated when given to an elderly patient.

5. List the responsibilities that the nurse has for drug orders in a nursing home that she does not have in an acute care area.

6. List several reasons why the elderly take more drugs than do younger members of our population.

ENVIRONMENTAL SAFETY PRECAUTIONS

Accidents, whether they cause serious injury to the elderly or not, and wherever they occur, have a profound effect upon the victim. They may precipitate a far more serious general breakdown of physical and mental health because of the elderly adult's precarious equilibrium. If an injury has occurred, the intense fear of reoccurrence may make the person reluctant to follow rehabilitative measures. There may be a tendency to lose independence in a trade for security.

All of the safety factors that are applicable with any patient are essential in caring for the elderly patient, plus those specifically necessary for special problems. These special problems include slowed reaction time, weakness, arthritic changes, failing vision and hearing, possible confusion, and side effects of medication.

Danger Areas

The Bathroom

The largest number of accidental falls seem to occur in the bathroom, on stairs, and in the kitchen in homes. In long-term care facilities, falls in the bathroom are the most common.

Bathing is safer in showers, preferably with a nonslip sitting arrangement and with nonslip floors. In some instances, a flexible-hose shower spray is preferred. When the patient is unable to shower himself, a shower chair that can be wheeled into the shower stall is used. If shower chairs are used, extreme care should be used to provide adequate covering for the patient, both for warmth and privacy. A safety strap should also be used on the chair.

Conventional tubs can be converted for safety for those able to use them. A tub seat, grab rails, and a shower spray can be added, as well as nonslip materials for the bottom of the tub. These adhesive strips are inappropriate, however, for institutional communal tubs, as the surface cannot be cleaned adequately.

The elevated bathtubs found furnished in health-care facilities are manufactured for the nurses' convenience. They are intended to be used with a pneumatic lift device, such as the "Hoyer" lift. Specific patients, particularly those with skin problems or those unable to sit in a shower chair, benefit from this total immersion. The anxiety and fright that this may cause in some patients must be weighed against the end results. Much of the anxiety has probably stemmed from improper handling at some point, or by previous experience with falls. Nursing personnel must be instructed carefully in the use of the lift, and each nurse should play the role of a patient and be dangled over a tub to fully appreciate the patient's anxiety. Collapsible rubber tubs are also available. These can be placed on carts and are especially useful when caring for the paraplegic patient.

Careful explanation of the procedure, regardless of the number of times it has been done, and slow, deliberate movements will do much to overcome the fears of the patient. If these fears cannot be calmed, and every bath causes great anxiety, tub baths should be discontinued, regardless of other advantages.

The Bedroom

The use of any loose rugs should be eliminated in the elderly person's environment; such usage in long-term care facilities violates state and federal safety regulations. Well-meaning friends and family who are not aware of these regulations need explanations if they bring in rugs to spare the elderly person the contact with cold floors. The ambulatory elderly person should wear shoes that fit well and support the foot, rather than soft slippers, which tend to slip or to come off.

Upon admission to the institution, the ambulatory patient should have a careful orientation to his living area, particularly his own room. A night light that illuminates the floor will be helpful, particularly if he must be up during the night. It is a good policy to leave the light on all night in the adjoining bathroom, for confusion during the dark hours is common and may lead to falls. If the beds have hand cranks, be sure they are not left out of their sockets, for serious bruises and falls can result from tripping against them.

The bedfast patient should always have his side rails up, as well as any patient who has a sedative at night or who is confused. After bedside care is given, the bed must always be left in the lowest position possible. The call bell should be securely attached to the bed linen in a position that can be easily reached by the patient.

Any type of electrical appliance, such as radios, shavers, or hair dryers should be checked by the facility engineer prior to use by the patient or nurse. In addition, all lamps, machines, appliances, or signal devices should be checked on a routine basis for frayed cords.

Communal electric shavers should not be used, as there is no safe method of cleaning them and preventing cross infections between patients.

Drugs and Other Dangerous Substances

Regardless of nursing principles, there is always the temptation to leave medication at the bedside of alert patients when they do not wish to take it immediately. It is especially dangerous in nursing homes to do so. There are always some confused persons present, and they may take medication other than their own with serious or fatal results. No medications should be kept on the bedside table for the same reason. Families should be informed of this policy for the safety of all.

No utility room where patients may enter should contain any germicidal solutions, cleaning compounds, or such materials except in locked cupboards. All patients must be protected, regardless of the small risk factor. Medications and poisons that may be accessible to patients may be used in suicide attempts.

Constant vigilance for locked medicine rooms and medicine carts is imperative. When medications are being passed, the cart should never be left unattended unless locked. These precautionary warnings seem redundant, as each student has heard them countless times. It is well to remember that only one lapse of caution can have serious results.

Wheelchairs

Patients who are not ambulatory and spend time in wheelchairs have special safety needs. The wheelchair should be inspected periodically

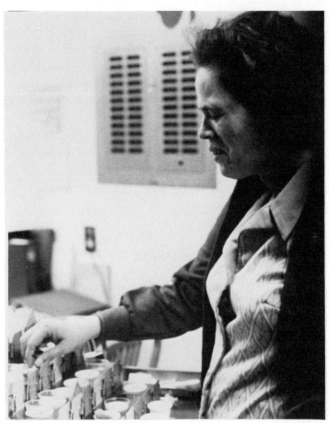

Photographer: Doris Wilson, RN
Model: Loretta A. Soper

The unattended medication cart may be a temptation to some patients.

for safety features. Brakes should function properly, and footrests should be sturdy and easily adjusted. If the patient is at all confused, prone to fall asleep easily, or has balance problems, safety belts should be in place. Shoulder "Posey" restraints are necessary with some patients. These restraints can be used for either minimum or maximum restraining power. The intent should be fully understood by the nurse. Any type of safety belt or restraint should be observed frequently for comfort. The ability of patients to maneuver their bodies regardless of safety belts is unbelievable, and patients may be so skillful that these maneuvers may result in injuries.

Placing a patient in a wheelchair with a safety belt or restraint does not release the nurse of constant responsibility for his safety

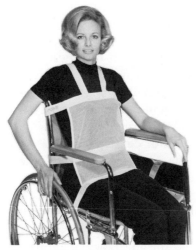 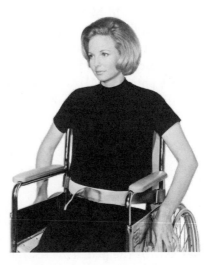

Courtesy of J. T. Posey Co.

A variety of restraints are available that assure the safety and comfort of the wheelchair patient.

and comfort. Patients who spend hours in wheelchairs should never be left in their rooms, but should be where they can easily be seen by nursing personnel. Their positions should be changed frequently if they are able to do so, or by the nurse if they are not able. Pressure areas, resulting in decubiti, can result from inactivity in wheelchairs as well as in beds. A bell or signal cord should be within easy reach of the wheelchair patient so that he can call for assistance as desired.

Other Restraints

The use of any restraint in a nursing home should be a last resort nursing measure. If the patient is agitated enough to require them, and if he is in danger of harming himself or others, a thorough assessment, which includes vital signs, medication review, and an examination for any external trauma should be made to attempt to ascertain the cause of agitation, if possible. Communication with the patient is essential to verbally explore the causes of his anxiety.

Chest restraints made of a woven material that can be cut with a scissors in case of emergency and where the arms can be moved freely, are the preferred type. Extreme care should be used so that the straps are tied securely to the bed frame, out of reach of the patient.

Restraints should be removed at least every six hours, so the patient can be ambulated or sat up. Turning from side to side should be done at least every two hours. This activity increases circulation.

The pelvic restraint is probably superior to the chest restraint for most patients. A restraint can be quickly made in an emergency by folding two separate bed sheets diagonally (long part of sheet). One sheet is placed under the pelvic region, and one over. The ends of the sheets are twisted until the body is firmly encased, with care that the free movement of the chest is not constricted. The ends of the sheet are brought underneath the bed and tied firmly to the frame.

A commercial variety of the pelvic restraint is available. When using this, the short strap is fastened to the bed frame, the longer is threaded through the slot in back of the pad and then secured to the other side of the bed. This restraint has the advantage of allowing the patient to sit up in bed and move about with more freedom than other types of restraints.

In cases of extreme agitation, restraints are contraindicated, as they increase anxiety. These patients should be transferred to an acute care facility that is equipped with a psychiatric unit to care for patients with this type of behavior. Restraints must not be used rou-

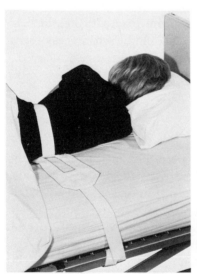 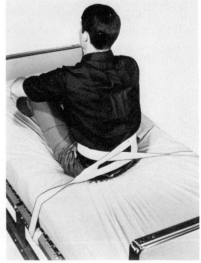

Courtesy of J. T. Posey Co.
Pelvic restraints are safe, comfortable, and reliable when correctly applied, as shown in these side and back views.

tinely nor be regarded as a normal nursing procedure. Communication and constant sensory stimulation will help eliminate confusion and agitation in all but a few instances.

Restraints, except for emergency safety measures, should not be used without a doctor's order, and then only when all other alternatives have been exhausted. Restraints should not be used as a punitive measure, and should not be seen as a measure to relieve nurses of using other alternatives of care. Each facility has its own policies concerning restraints, and the nurse must be fully aware of these policies. Nursing notes should indicate when the patient's behavior that necessitated restraints began, what measures were taken to alleviate it, and the results of these efforts. In addition, notes should indicate when restraints were applied, the type, when they were released, and any other nursing measures concerned with the restraints and the patient's reaction to them.

Burns

Elderly peoples' sense of touch is less sensitive to heat; therefore the they are more prone to burns. The use of hot water bottles and heating pads should not be permitted in an institutional setting. Their use in homes should be discouraged, particularly for the elderly diabetic. Such appliances for external heat as the "Aqua-K" pads are permissible, as the heat is constant and cannot be applied when it is too hot.

Nursing personnel must always be alert for compliance to smoking policies, as the danger of fire in beds is particularly high with the elderly. Usually specific areas of the facility, outside of the bedrooms, are designated for smoking; unless someone is in constant attendance while the patient smokes, if the patient is unable to leave the bedroom.

The hot-water supply in homes or facilities for elderly persons should never be over 110° and should be automatically controlled to decrease the possibility of burns by scalding.

Assisting with Ambulation

Many elderly adults are constantly in fear of falling and, as a result, are reluctant to leave their beds or chairs. This fear can be so pronounced that toileting, eating, and socializing are neglected. These

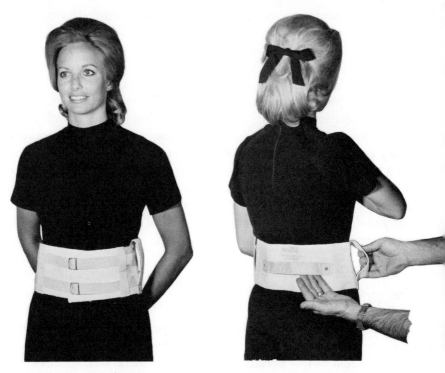

Courtesy of F. T. Posey Co.

Front and back views of transfer or ambulation belt.

people must be aroused to change position and to reduce isolation. The fear of falling and/or the difficulties encountered in assisting some persons to move can be greatly simplified by the use of a transfer belt. A transfer or ambulation belt should be washable and sturdy, made of nonstretch material. It should have a dependable buckle or be long enough for a square knot to be made.

The belt is secured around the patient's waist, and the nurse grasps it at the back or sides. If the patient begins to slip, the motion is easily halted. If it is necessary to allow the patient to be lowered to the floor, the movement is easily controlled to prevent trauma to either patient or nurse. These belts can be used in a number of one- and two-man transfer techniques, and are safer and less harmful than grasping the patient's body.

Other Aids to Ambulation

All hallways in long-term care facilities must have handrails to assist patients in walking. The rails serve as a security measure for those who are unsteady, weak, have problems of equilibrium, or have poor vision.

Poor vision or confusion also make it difficult for some persons to identify their rooms, the elevator door, or bathrooms. Many simple devices can assist these people to find their way easily. Brightly colored wool tassels, pictures, raised emblems, or other objects that can be distinguished by touch or sight are most helpful. The patient

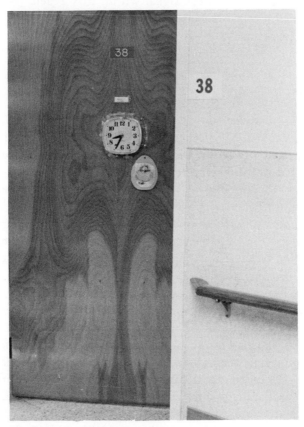

Photographer: Doris Wilson, RN

Simple devices make it easier for the confused or visually handicapped patient to find his room.

is spared the indignity of asking assistance each time or wandering about aimlessly.

Signal Devices

Each bed must have a signal device readily available for the patient to summon assistance. All bathrooms and shower rooms should also be furnished with them. Constant monitoring to see that the cords and signals are in good working order is imperative. Bed patients must never be left without their call bells. After bed making is done, it is easy to forget to reattach the signal within easy reach. (Needless to say, the availability of a signal is useless unless its summons is responded to quickly.)

Emergencies

All health care institutions have written disaster plans, to be used in case of fire, explosion, or other disasters. The segment for fire safety includes planned fire drills and periodic inspections of the building by fire marshals or other fire department personnel.

At intervals, nursing and other personnel are alerted by fire drills, and all staff members learn the proper procedures for the eventuality of a fire plus their own specific role in the emergency. Patients, who are the object of the instruction and the practice, are rarely included in these drills and may never have any direction given to them concerning their own behavior in an emergency. Many are capable of helping themselves and others.

Each patient who is capable of understanding should be instructed periodically about what will be done in case of fire and what he can do to assist. Anyone who has had any explanation is more likely to cooperate than if he is totally unaware of what is being done to save him. Even patients who have problems of communication can be prepared to some extent. Each nursing care plan cardex should be clearly labeled to make it easy to identify which patients will need to be removed by wheelchair, blanket carry, or stretcher. Those patients with communication problems should be identified. All fire alarms should have auditory and visual signals, to include those who are hard of hearing.

The instruction may be disturbing, but the knowledge that fires cause unnecessary deaths each year in such health care facilities should mitigate the temporary anxiety of patients. Including them in plans as responsible adults may also be beneficial to their self-esteem.

THE ADMINISTRATION OF DRUGS TO THE ELDERLY

Eighty-six percent of the population suffer one or more chronic diseases as they reach 65 years of age. Their need for prescription drugs is three times more than all other age groups combined (Haran, 1978, p. 57). One of the major factors in the prolongation of life has been the introduction of drugs that cure or alleviate problems that in earlier days caused death. Some drugs simply make old age more comfortable. These drugs do not cure old age, and not all are lifesavers. When they are used incorrectly, they can be lethal. The elderly, who comprise 10 percent of our population, take 25 percent of all prescription drugs each year (Basen, 1977, p. 43). This follows the trend of our culture, which seems to demand a pill for every discomfort.

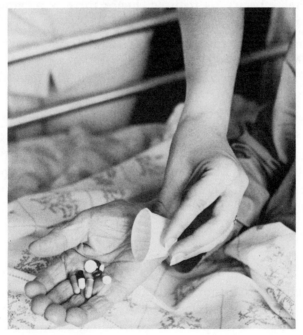

Photographer: Doris Wilson, RN

Poly-pharmacy—a potential danger to the elderly patient.

Katchthaler and associates, in a study of 100 elderly patients, found that the average number of drugs taken daily was 3.33, the average number of pills was 6.34 daily. Seventy-three percent of the patients took 3 drugs daily, 44 percent took 4, and 22 percent took 5 drugs. This multiplicity of drugs has been labeled "poly-pharmacy," which is defined as a concurrent prescription of several different drugs in dosages or frequencies higher than those known to be therapeutically necessary (Katchthaler, et al, 1977, p. 308).

The changes that occur in the elderly have been discussed in earlier chapters; these changes can be summarized as they influence the reactions of the elderly adult to his medication as follows:

1. Because of reduced activity, arteriosclerosis, venous stasis, and reduced cardiac output, circulation to the cells is diminished. This results in a decrease of both oxygen and nutrition to the cells.

2. Because of the above, pulmonary capacity is reduced. The amount of air that can be expelled following full inspiration (vital capacity) is reduced, hence there is retention of carbon dioxide in the lungs.

3. The decreased cardiac output also results in decreased circulation to the kidneys. Decreased filtration ability of the kidney results in a decreased ability to detoxify drugs and other toxic substances.

4. Decreased circulation results in decreased ability to properly absorb, use, and break down medications.

5. The elderly person has less reserve cardiac ability, resulting in a loss of the body's ability to maintain homeostasis. Thus, stress is not easily overcome, and the ability to function in overcoming drug reactions is greatly reduced.

Drug Knowledge in the Elderly

Elderly adults who are not institutionalized may suffer many unforeseen reactions to their drugs. While the prescribing physician may alert his patient to the possibilities of some, other reactions are so unpredictable that they are not anticipated. While some reactions will be reported by the patient and changes made in the prescriptions, it is unknown how many untoward reactions are attributed to "part of growing old," and cause more problems than were originally present. The number of fatalities or admissions to health care facilities resulting from drug-induced symptoms is unknown.

One of the major questions to be asked in assessing whether the elderly adult is taking his medication as ordered is, "What is his visual ability to read labels?" Another question frequently asked by nurses is whether the person can read at all. Labels on prescriptions are typed, and the size of the label may be next to impossible to read for a person with failing vision. In the majority of cases, no question concerning visual acuity is made by the pharmacist, nor is repetition of the doctor's orders concerning the amount of drug and its prescribed frequency made. Larger print on labels would be beneficial, as would careful explanations of the directions pertinent to the drug.

Other causes of misuse of drugs due to lack of information and instruction are as follows:

1. Overdosage
2. Self-selection of drugs
3. Omitting medication
4. Medications duplicated by prescription from a different physician
5. The prescription indicates "as needed," which is vague and misunderstood
6. Drugs for similar complaints are exchanged with others
7. Outdated drugs are used
8. Automatic refills may allow overdosage
9. Prescription medication is inappropriate for the patient
10. Prescription was the result of telephone communication
11. Patient was too confused to use medication correctly

(Basen, 1977, p. 43)

Drug Systems

The patient in a long-term care facility may be no better cared for in his drug therapy program than if he is taking his own medications at home. Unless the nursing home is connected with an acute care facility or is very large (200–300 beds), usually no pharmacist is employed in the institution. Doctor's orders for medications are filled by a local pharmacy or pharmacies. Patients in the nursing home have the freedom of choice of where their medications will be purchased, unless they are welfare recipients. The patient's drug orders are reviewed at least monthly by a pharmacy consultant in the facility.

On his monthly visit, the consultant, with his "patient profiles" (a complete list of all of the medications ordered by the physician for each patient) and with information concerning the patient's age, weight, general condition, and known allergies, evaluates the facility's drug system. He will check such records as medication sheets, nurses' notes, and laboratory tests (if applicable). This review of the patient's drug regimen (all drugs, both prescription and nonprescription, that are ordered by the physician, includes PRN medications on order but not recently used) is conducted to find any irregularities. Irregularities are anything contrary to what is usual, proper, accepted, or right in drug administration. Irregularities also include drug administration errors, questionable interpretation of physician's orders by nursing staff, and adverse drug reactions and interactions.

The consultant provides the facility with documentation that he has reviewed each patient's regimen. Any irregularities are reported for correction. Nursing responsibilities include having the records easily available to the consultant and clarifying notes on the patients' records as necessary.

Each month, the nursing service department sends the attending physician a form on each of his patients, which lists the current drugs, his vital signs, and any recommendations for drug changes, deletions, or requests for other drugs based upon his current status. To renew or change any drug, the physician reviews the list and recommendations, signs the form, and returns it to the facility. If the doctor has visited his patient within the month and reviewed his orders, this postal exchange is not necessary.

Ordering drugs by review imposes a greatly increased responsibility on the nurse. These drugs are being given to a group of patients taking higher than average varieties of medications, with increased risk of reactions. The margin for clerical errors of dosage and frequency has been shown to be high, as these orders may be recopied a number of times.

The presence of drug reference texts on the nursing units is of great assistance to the nurse, but they are not organized for rapid referral and contain a wealth of information to plow through for the answers desired. The volume of medications to be given at a specific time is itself a deterrent to seeking information about drugs.

In some long-term facilities, in-service classes on medications or related subjects will be offered by the pharmacy consultant, but this opportunity is not widely available.

Many medication systems are available to insure the safe, quick administration and charting of drugs. In some facilities, the outdated, error-prone medication card system is still utilized. A system where the medications are assembled for each patient from the patient's drug list, and the medication's administration is charted on the same form, results in time saving, less duplication of records, and a higher degree of accuracy. No drug system is perfect, and nurses can change it to be more efficient. In most instances, the only excuse for not changing a system that has outlived its usefulness is habit.

The unit-dose system also reduces error, but at this time the cost per dose is greater than other packaging methods, and it is used more frequently in large metropolitan area facilities. Regardless of the system used, the same safeguards are applicable as those used in acute care areas.

Patient Reactions to Drugs

Some of the changes of structure and function that occur with aging have been discussed. These changes can alter, weaken, or strengthen the normal actions of drugs.

The absorption, circulation throughout the body, metabolism, and excretion of drugs is altered in the geriatric patient as shown in Table 7-1.

Some drugs that frequently cause problems when given to the elderly are listed in Table 7-2. Close observations for side effects must be made and their occurrence communicated to the registered nurse, to the physician, and to peers orally and by notations on the patient's record and medication list.

The nurse must constantly evaluate the medications that the patient receives, not only for untoward reactions, but for adequate

TABLE 7-1

Common Physiological Changes and the Possible Result in Drug Action

Physiological Changes	Possible Result in Drug Action
Body weight, fluid ↓ K ↓ Na ↑	Drug overdose
Cardiac reserve ↓ Cardiac output ↓ Venous congestion ↑ O_2 absorption ↓ O_2 exchange ↓	Drugs not completely adsorbed, uneven body distribution
Glomerular filtration ↓ and absorption Excretion ↓ Renal blood flow ↓	Retention of drugs Drug intoxication
Liver function ↓	Impaired detoxification and metabolism

dosage levels. The need to reduce or discontinue the drug may also be included in the monthly drug resume forwarded to the physician. The nurse should always base her recommendations upon the following:

1. The patient should receive the least amount of drugs possible, based upon his primary symptoms and diagnosis.
2. All drugs should be considered potentially dangerous and given in the smallest dosages possible to produce results.

When the physician reduces the amount of or discontinues a drug that is no longer necessary, which reduces the number of pills the person receives, this often results in a problem. Many elderly adults have placed great confidence in their medications and know the exact number, color, and time they are due. The loss of a pill because of the physician's order can severely upset their security and may result in a verbal attack upon the nurse, regardless of careful and repeated explanations. It is particularly difficult to explain to the patient that this is what the doctor has ordered when the patient may not have seen the doctor for a number of weeks.

TABLE 7-2
Drugs to be Used with Caution by the Elderly

The pharmaceutical agents listed here may require dosage adjustment and/or special precautions when prescribed for elderly outpatients, particularly those who live alone.
(This list was prepared by Barry Greenberg, PharmD, New Haven, Conn.)

Analgesics/antipyretics

indomethacin (Indocin)
morphine sulfate
opiates
oxyphenbutazone (Oxalid, Tandearil)
pentazocine HCl (Talwin HCl)
phenylbutazone (Azolid, Butazolidin)
salicylates

Antibiotics/antimicrobials

aminoglycoside antibiotics*†:
    gentamicin sulfate (Garamycin)
    kanamycin sulfate (Kantrex)
    neomycin sulfate (Mycifradin
        Sulfate, Neobiotic)
    streptomycin sulfate
colistimethate sodium (Coly-Mycin M)†
nalidixic acid (NegGram)
nitrofurantoin (Cyantin, etc.)
sulfonamides, long-acting:
    sulfadimethoxine (Madribon)
    sulfameter (Sulla)
    sulfamethoxypyridazine (Midicel)
tetracycline HCl and tetracycline
    derivatives

Anticholinergics

atropine and related compounds

Anticoagulants

bishydroxycoumarin (Dicumarol)
heparin sodium† (Panheprin, etc.)

sodium warfarin (Coumadin,
    Panwarfin)

Antidepressants

CNS stimulants:
    dextroamphentamine sulfate
        (Dexedrine)
    methylphenidate HCl (Ritalin HCl)
MAO inhibitors:
    isocarboxazid (Marplan)
    nialamide (Niamid)
    phenelzine (Nardil)
    tranylcypromine (Parnate)
Tricyclic antidepressants:
    amitriptyline HCl (Elavil HCl)
    desipramine HCl (Norpramin,
        Pertofrane)
    doxepin HCl (Adapin, Sinequan)
    imipramine HCl (Presamine,
        Tofranil)
    nortriptyline HCl (Aventyl HCl)
    protriptyline HCl (Vivactil HCl)

Antihypertensives

guanethidine (Ismelin)
hydralazine (Apresoline)
methyldopa (Aldomet)
pargyline (Eutonyl)
reserpine (Rau-Sed, Reserpoid, etc.)
rauwolfia serpentina (Hyperloid, etc.)

—————— *(Continued)* ——————

*If renal function is diminished
†Primarily used in the hospitalized patient
SOURCE: From *Nursing Update*, "Is that Problem Drug Related?" (October 1975): 1ff.

TABLE 7-2
Drugs to be Used with Caution by the Elderly (Cont.)

Cathartics	Oral hypoglycemics

Cathartics

mineral oil, saline cathartics, etc.

Digitalis glycosides

digitalis leaf* (Digitora, Pil-Digis, etc.)
digitoxin (Crystodigin, Purodigin, etc.)
digoxin* (Davoxin, Lanoxin)

Diuretics

chlorthalidone (Hygroton)
ethacrynic acid (Edecrin)
furosemide (Lasix)
thiazides:
   bendroflumethiazide (Naturetin)
   benzthiazide (Aquatag, etc.)
   chlorothiazide (Diuril)
   cyclothiazide (Anhydron)
   hydrochlorothiazide (Hydrodiuril,
     Esidrix, Oretic)
   hydroflumethiazide (Saluron)
   methyclothiazide (Enduron)
   polythiazide (Renese)
   trichlormethiazide (Metahydrin,
     Naqua)
triamterene (Dyrenium)

Oral hypoglycemics

sulfonylureas:
   acetohexamide (Dymelor)
   chlorpropamide (Diabinese)
   tolazamide (Tolinase)
   tolbutamide (Orinase)

Sedatives/tranquilizers

barbiturates
chlorprothixene HCl (Taractan)
haloperidol (Haldol)
minor tranquilizers:
   chlordiazepoxide HCl (Librium)
   clorazepate dipotassium (Tranxene)
   diazepam (Valium)
   flurazepam HCl (Dalmane)
   oxazepam (Serax)
phenothiazines (Compazine, etc.)
thiothixene (Navane, Navaron)

Steroids/hormones

cortisone and glucocorticosteroids
liothyronine sodium (Cytomel)
testosterone

    Continued reassurance concerning medications and changes in medications are necessary for the patient's feeling of security. Sometimes only time will erase the anger and frustration of the patient. If the nurse will assure the patient that newly ordered medications will only be used for as short a period as necessary for one specific problem, the patient may be more understanding of changes made in his drug regimen.

    The physician and the nurse must communicate and work together to assure that the patient has the proper medications, but as few as is possible, and only for as long as actually needed. The nurse should not be frustrated if the doctor does not follow her recommendations. He is responsible for his drug orders and knows the patient and the total situation of the patient. He must learn to trust the nurse's judgment, based on her knowledge and past behavior.

ASEPTIC SAFETY PRECAUTIONS

Any health-care institution is envisioned by the public as one that not only safeguards the patient's present condition but enhances it.

Nosocomial infections are those that originate in a health-care institution. Every precaution must be taken so that these infections do not occur. The patients normally present in a long-term care facility are particularly susceptible to infection because they usually have a variety of health problems already present, they may have nutritional deficiencies, and they do not have the strength and vigor of younger persons to resist diseases.

Bacteriologic safety is the elimination of disease-producing organisms and the dirt that harbors them in a manner that does not harm the patient nor cause cross infection or reinfection. All departments in the facility must be informed about proper care procedures and cleaning techniques.

In the past thirty years, health care has focused more on curing diseases than on preventing infection. This trend has resulted in strains of organisms that are drug resistant. We must work to prevent infection rather than assume they can all be cured once contracted.

Long-term care facilities employ many nursing assistants who are not required to have a background of scientific knowledge. It is the responsibility, therefore, of the practical nurse, as well as the registered nurse, to see that all perform their duties using good aseptic techniques.

Thorough hand washing is the one most important activity to combat infection. Hands must always be washed between caring for different patients and prior to starting any nursing procedure.

Some of the most common examples of violations of medical asepsis observable in long-term care facilities are as follows:

Linen Handling

1. Throwing soiled bed linen on the floor or on a chair after removal from the bed. The floor is grossly contaminated, and the linen picks up additional organisms, leaving some on the floor. Laundry does not sterilize linens; it only cleans them.

2. Shaking linen when placing it on or removing it from the bed, adding to airborne bacteria and lint.

3. Using facecloths to clean the patient after a bowel movement instead of first using toilet tissue.

4. Carrying linen to a receptacle clutched to the body, thereby grossly contaminating the uniform.

5. Removing unused linen to a linen closet or cart after it has been in a patient's room.

6. Nursing personnel should never be allowed or required to sort linen in preparation for washing nor be involved in any laundry procedures. Grossly soiled linens should never be rinsed by nursing personnel. These activities all result in gross contamination of the nurse (and her uniform), who, despite careful hand washing, will endanger the patient and her peers.

Communal Use of Articles

1. Using electric shavers from patient to patient should not be permitted, as there is no efficient method to clean these appliances between patients.

2. Use of communal soap in showers or bath. Soap does harbor bacteria.

3. When shower chairs are used for all patients, the chair must be cleaned after each patient's use with disinfectant. The constant wetting in showers does not clean this article on which people sit with the perineal area in contact with the chair. Particular attention should be given to the underside of the chair, which may be found grossly contaminated with feces.

4. Some wheelchairs are used for a variety of patients, and persons with urinary and fecal incontinence sit in them for hours. A cleaning routine after each use must be established.

5. Hoyer lift slings should not be used interchangeably. If the woven-material type is used, each patient using the sling should have his own, which would be laundered periodically. If the waterproof-plastic type of sling is used, it should be cleaned with a disinfectant agent following each use.

6. Bed scales should be thoroughly cleaned with a disinfectant between each use.

7. Each patient should have his own body lotion, bath powder, and toilet articles. They should never be placed in a "community" container that travels from bedside to bedside as it is used.
8. Signal-bell cords or television control cords should be thoroughly cleaned with disinfectants between patient bed occupancy. In addition, if the cords are dropped on the floor, they must be cleaned before being replaced on the patient's bed.

Long-term care facilities should include in their policy manuals specific measures to reduce or eliminate sources of infection and to break contact between the source of infection and the host. The measures most likely to control infections are:

1. Thorough hand washing.
2. Strict practice of medical aseptic technique by all personnel. Periodic review of the principles of asepsis conducted during in-service classes.
3. Strict practice of surgical asepsis when sterility is required.
4. Restriction from work of any employee who has a staphylococcal lesion or other infection, such as infected acne, boils, or inflamed throat with temperature.
5. Thorough ongoing and terminal disinfection of all materials and environment for all known or suspected cases of infectious nature.
6. Housekeeping and maintenance departments must use biological principles in their practices.
7. Effective pest control.
8. Sanitary food services.
9. Scrupulous cleanliness throughout the facility.

The nurse's role in prevention of infection is one of constant personal vigilance and supervision. Any potential dangers should be reported immediately. The elderly adult's balance between health and disease is always precarious.

The responsibility for cleaning of multiple-use equipment cannot always be relegated to the housekeeping department. If patient care is to proceed in an orderly manner, some cleaning will inevitably fall to the nurse and be part of the safe care she gives her patient.

REVIEW QUESTIONS

1. Why are special safety precautions necessary when caring for elderly persons?
2. What steps are necessary before restraints are applied?
3. What precautions are necessary after restraints are applied?
4. Why does the nurse have greater responsibilities for medications in a long-term care facility than in an acute care area?
5. Name some hazards you might encounter with dangerous substances in a nursing facility.
6. What changes take place in the body of the elderly adult that affect the results of medications?

RECOMMENDED ACTIVITIES

1. Survey one nursing unit and identify safety hazards. As a class, make recommendations to eradicate the hazards.
2. With a fellow student, practice lowering each other over a bed or bathtub. What were your feelings about the procedure?
3. Count the number of medications and the number of pills necessary for a 24-hour period for your elderly patient. Does this number agree with the research quoted in the text?
4. With a fellow student, observe such areas as patient bathrooms, shower rooms, utility rooms and medicine room. Describe in class any violations in asepsis. Also describe some measures utilized that helped maintain good technique.

BIBLIOGRAPHY

Basen, Michele. "The Elderly and Drugs—Problem Overview and Program Strategy." *Public Health Reports* 92 (January/February, 1977): 43.

Brown, Martha et al. "Drug-Drug Interactions among Residents in Homes for the Elderly." *Nursing Research* 26 (January/February 1977): 47-52.

Brady, W.S. *Drugs and the Elderly*. University of Southern California, Los Angeles: Ethel Percy Andrus Gerontology Center, 1975, p. 1-6.

Combs, K.L. "Staying Well While Growing Old: Preventative Care in the Elderly," Part 3. *American Journal of Nursing* 78 (August 1978): 1339-1341.

Feist, R.R. "A Survey of Accidental Falls in a Small Home for the Aged." *Journal of Gerontological Nursing* 4 (November/December 1978): 15-17.

Gotz, Bridget E. and Vincent P. "Drugs and the Elderly." *American Journal of Nursing* 78 (August 1978): 1347-1349.

Haran, Zachary I. "Geriatric Medications: How the Aged Are Hurt by Drugs Meant to Help." *RN* (November 1977): pp. 40-57.

Hicks, H. et al. "Patients' Medication Profile Keeps the Records Straight." *Hospital Formulary* 13 (January 1978): 58-60.

Jenkins, Betty L. "A Case Against Sleepers." *Journal of Geontological Nursing* 2 (March/April 1976): 10-13.

Klabak, Loraine. "Getting a Grip on the Transfer Belt Technique." *Nursing 1978* 8 (February 1978): 10.

Kalchthaler, Thomas et al. "Incidence of Polypharmacy in a Long-term Care Facility." *Journal of the American Geriatric Society* 24 (July 1977): 308-313.

McLennan, William. "Dangerous Drugs." *Nursing Times*, July 15, 1976.

Pablo, R.Y. "Patient Accidents in Long-Term-Care Facilities." *Canadian Journal of Public Health*, May/June 1977.

Sehested, P. et al. "Falls by Hospitalized Elderly Patients: Causes, Prevention." *Geriatrics* 32 (April 1977): 101-108.

Smith, Cynthia. "Accidents and the Elderly." *Nursing Times*, December 2, 1976.

_____. "Is that Problem Drug Related? *Nursing Update* 6 (October 1975): 5.

chapter 8

Nutritional Needs of the Elderly Adult

OBJECTIVES

After studying this unit, the student will be able to:

1. List three reasons for caloric reduction in the diet of the elderly adult.

2. Identify the basic four food groups and give examples of foods in each group.

3. Explain why dietary supplements are unnecessary in normal diets.

4. Describe three reasons why changes in dietary habits are difficult.

5. Discuss two advantages to the elderly of portable or communal meals.

6. Explain why sodium restrictions are necessary in some diets.

161

America has developed a superior food growing, packaging, and distribution industry. We also possess a wealth of nutritional knowledge. None of this assures all of our citizens of good nutrition. The elderly, who have less access to knowledge and generally less money to spend, have increased problems with nutrition. Poorly balanced diets are particularly serious to the elderly because they accelerate aging and deterioration by complicating any existing physical or mental problems.

SPECIFIC NUTRITIONAL NEEDS

As the individual ages, there is gradual loss of cellular function, as well as some reduction in general activity level. Because of the reduction in demand, the need for calories is also reduced approximately 7.5 percent for every decade past 25 years. As everyone has a truly distinctive activity level, there is no standard caloric requirement that will fit each person. After 50 years of age, the total caloric allowance for a man is approximately 2,400 calories and for a woman, 1,800 calories. The most accurate criteria for caloric intake is the maintenance of normal weight.

The basic diet (Table 8-1) depicts the daily requirements of essential nutrients. As the person ages, the amount of calories he should consume in addition to these essential requirements is gradually lowered.

The Meat Group

The amount of protein required per kilogram of body weight for all adults over 25 years of age is 0.8 grams. This requirement does not

163

TABLE 8-1
Food and Nutrition Board, National Academy of Sciences–National Research Council
Recommended Daily Dietary Allowances, Revised 1973

| | (years) | Weight | | Height | | Energy | Protein | Fat-Soluble Vitamins | | | |
| | From Up to | (kg) | (lbs) | (cm) | (in) | (Δ cal) | (g) | Vitamin A Activity | | Vitamin D | Vitamin C Activity |
								(RE)	(IU)	(IU)	(IU)
Males	51+	70	154	172	69	2400	56	1,000	5,000		15
Females	51+	58	128	162	65	1800	46	800	4,000		12

| | Water-Soluble Vitamins | | | | | | | Minerals | | | | | |
	Ascorbic Acid (mg)	Folacin (μg)	Niacin (mg)	Ribo-flavin (mg)	Thia-min (mg)	Vita-min B_6 (mg)	Vita-min B_{12} (μg)	Calcium (mg)	Phos-phorus (mg)	Iodine (μg)	Iron (mg)	Magnesium (mg)	Zinc (mg)
Males	45	400	16	1.5	1.2	2.0	3.0	800	800	110	10	350	15
Females	45	400	12	1.1	1.0	2.0	3.0	800	800	80	10	300	15

alter, regardless of one's age. About one-fourth to one-half of the total protein should be of animal source, the remainder should be of plant origin. Meats, fish, poultry, eggs or cheese can be supplemented by dry beans, peas, or nuts.

Milk

The need for milk continues throughout life. Two glasses per day are recommended. Either cheese, ice cream, or other milk-made foods can supply part of the daily requirement. If there is any weight problem, low fat or skim milk is preferable.

Vegetables and Fruits

Although the exact total amount of carbohydrates necessary is unknown, 59 percent of the total calories should be in this group. These foods should be used for four servings each per day. The diet should include a dark-green leafy or deep-yellow vegetable or yellow fruit at least three to four times a week for Vitamin A. At least one serving each day of citrus fruit or tomatoes is required to supply Vitamin C.

Bread and Cereals

Bread and cereals should be chosen from enriched or whole grain products and four servings used per day. These foods provide iron, protein, several B vitamins, and food energy in the form of carbohydrates. If a sufficient amount of carbohydrates is not included in the diet, the protein intake will be utilized by the body for energy needs rather than for cellular repair and maintenance.

Fats

Fats provide energy, essential fatty acids, and fat soluble vitamins, and are usually included in the basic four food groups. About 20 percent of the diet should consist of fat, with an emphasis on polyunsaturated fats of plant origin. The usual sources of fat are meat, margarines, cooking oils, and butter.

FADS AND FANCIES

Each year drug, food, and cosmetic manufacturers spend millions of dollars promoting products that promise longevity, potency, retardation of aging, and a variety of wonderous results. Food fads cost the American public over one billion dollars annually. The elderly person, who observes changes taking place in his body, appearance, and energy level, is particularly susceptible to these extravagant claims. Some of the most common are as described below.

Amino Acid Supplements

Amino acid supplements are expensive and are unpalatable without the addition of other substances. They may be irritating to the gastrointestinal tract. If the diet includes milk, eggs, and meat (fish or poultry), additional amino acids are unnecessary. If the diet is lacking in essential amino acids, it should be corrected by the addition of natural foods. Only if there is a pathological problem and only on a doctor's prescription should amino acid supplements be given to an elderly person. Recent studies have shown that a high-protein diet that does not contain the other essential nutrient requirements can cause death when certain medical problems exist in the patient.

Vitamins

Special geriatric vitamin B complex preparations for the elderly are very popular. These "specially formulated" preparations are frequently more expensive than other vitamin B forms and many incorrectly indicate that the elderly have increased requirements for the vitamin. The need does not change during adulthood, although the individual's normal diet may not provide sufficient quantities for good nutrition. The use of any self-medication should always be discouraged. If the person has been ill, additional supplements may be ordered by the physician.

Laxatives

As the body's metabolism slows down, the peristaltic action and tonus is reduced, the bowel patterns of some elderly adults change as a result. Many people have an intensified concern about their bowel habits and purchase patent medications and special foods for regularity. The practical nurse should explain that having a daily bowel movement is not essential for good health. The nurse should teach the patient that daily enemas and prolonged use of laxatives are not wise because they may cause natural elimination reflexes to be lost. Many elderly adults choose diets that are smooth in texture, either from preference or because of lack of teeth or poor-fitting dentures. This type of diet further promotes poor elimination. Fluid intake, foods high in bulk, and activity should be increased when there is a bowel problem.

Minerals

In normal aging, additional minerals are not necessary if a balanced diet is being adhered to. Advertisements would have one believe that all elderly people need calcium and iron supplements. A poor diet may lack these minerals, particularly if the aged feel that milk is unnecessary in the diet. Studies do indicate that women of all ages have a 21 to 30 percent deficit in calcium intake. After menopause, iron deficiencies in women are no longer a problem.

Health Foods

A current fad is the health food store or restaurant. Specially packaged health foods are said to be "natural" or "organic" and are fertilized not by chemicals but by organic waste materials. If one is very knowledgeable about food content, meals from organic and vegetarian sources can be adequate and nutritious. Unless one has well-documented chemical allergies, such foods are not necessary for good health and are quite expensive.

Some foods are marketed as "diabetic foods" and are packed without sugar. These foods are more expensive and not always easily obtainable. If the diabetic patient is taught to use a food exchange list, there is no need for specially processed food. Food exchange lists are available from the American Diabetic Association and from most physicians and hospitals.

No single food or drug has unique health-giving powers. "Special" foods that claim to cure or rejuvenate appeal more to the emotions and vanity than to the intellect. Correct information about diet and understanding of the diet are important to the health of the elderly adult.

While faddism can never be completely halted because people continue to hope for miracles, national education and monitoring by the Food and Drug Administration can prevent false advertisement.

BARRIERS TO GOOD NUTRITION

Many elderly adults live on fixed incomes, which do not keep pace with inflation. While several raises in Social Security benefits have occurred, payments are from twelve to sixteen months behind the decline in purchasing power. The amount of money available for food and rent is very limited and is complicated by several factors, as follows:

1. Many of the elderly become poor after retirement and are not adept at changing their life-styles.
2. The present generation of elderly have a low educational average and do not always understand nutritional needs nor management of funds.
3. Many live in single rooms where storage and preparation of food is difficult or forbidden.
4. Specially prescribed diets may cause additional costs and may require more shopping and more preparation.
5. Food preparation and consumption habits of a lifetime are difficult to change.

When sufficient monies are available for food, fear of the future or a strong desire to leave something to heirs may cause the person to skimp on essential needs.

Old people are preyed upon by society at times. One striking example is a low-rent area in Arizona, served by small grocery stores that were convenient for the elderly and that routinely raised their prices the day before the mail delivery of Social Security checks. Many also charged fifty cents or more to cash the checks of these, their regular customers (Weber, 1972).

The elderly have a higher than average history of health problems that require constant medication. If the person is not on public assistance, the cost of medications takes a large chunk out of his budget. In some instances, a choice must be made between food or medicine. Elimination of either one speeds deterioration of health.

The use of food stamps, commodity foods, and other community services should be urged to assure that the individual is able to afford an adequate diet.

Availability of Shopping Facilities

The number and variety of stores in the United States is enormous, but the majority of them are constructed and situated for access by automobile. After age 65, the number of persons who have cars and those who retain drivers' licenses declines with each additional year of age. If the elderly live in small towns where the traffic patterns are simple, they can usually remain mobile longer. In more densely populated areas, where congested freeways are present, the rate drops. The day of the neighborhood grocery is almost gone, except for small quick-service markets where the choice of merchandise is limited and prices may be double those available elsewhere. Whether the elderly adult drives or arrives at a large shopping area by bus, it may be almost impossible for him to walk the long distances required from the parking lots. Transportation within shopping centers has been almost totally ignored, and shopping centers remain the domain of the younger, more vigorous citizen.

Many old people utilize taxi service for grocery buying, which is an expensive mode of transportation, but which may have the added advantage of the generous driver who will usually carry purchases to the door. The lack of public transportation nationwide has been publicized for years, with little improvement, and with a continued increase of private automobiles. Mobility may be as important to good diet as knowledge of the right foods and the money with which to purchase it.

SOCIAL AND CULTURAL CONSIDERATIONS OF DIET

Attitudes about Food

Changing any long-term behavior is difficult. An attempt to change eating habits is very hard, as eating is an activity as unique and as important to the individual as one's sexual habits. Eating is not just a necessity for maintaining life but is a reflection of the total background of the person—his environment, religion, and ethnic identity. Disturbance of lifelong habits can result in stress, anger, and depression.

The difficulty of changing eating habits can be judged by the number of people who go on reducing diets and lose weight, only to go back to old habits and regain weight time after time.

The present generation of elderly adults lived through years of the depression, which made a profound impression on many, particularly in matters of food. Food servings had to be eaten with no waste. Perhaps this memory is especially discouraging when portions served to elderly persons are too large for lagging appetites, so nothing is eaten because of feelings of defeat and guilt.

Food is closely tied to distinct memories of life and the food and pleasure of past moments are interwoven. A patient in a southwestern nursing home related to a nurse, "Oh, I remember the Christmas Eves we had! Years ago it was a fast day, and we always had green-corn tamales and a big decorated cake—it was our Dad's birthday too . . . ." An eighty-four-year-old lady said, "I hate whole baked ham—they always remind me of funerals. I feel like I'm choking if I eat it." This was said when the nursing home served ham rather than turkey on Thanksgiving. Another patient said, "I remember the first fresh peas— we shelled them—all us kids on the front veranda. When Ma cooked them, we ate huge servings—some of us got sick. In a few days we couldn't stand peas. They just don't taste that good now, and all my brothers and sisters are gone. . . ."

Professional caretakers sometimes want to completely revise eating habits in the attempt to improve normal diets or to teach new therapeutic diets to patients. No diet is completely incorrect, and if the current eating patterns are closely assessed, the necessary changes may be very few. Little alterations are more readily accepted and more closely adhered to than sudden complete revisions. In any change, if the action is to be successful, the person must understand why change is necessary. This can best be accomplished by full explanations of the need for change by a team approach: the doctor, nurse and dietitian, and significant others. As the person becomes aware of the need, teaching can begin. As the revised diet is served, continued explanation of the reasons for specific foods as well as praise for conformity to the new diet should be given.

In reviewing the interrelatedness of food to the total makeup of personality, it is clear that this or any change, especially radical change, will create stress in the elderly person. The importance of proper diet in recovering from illness and in the maintenance of well being may be of more consequence than any medication or treatment. The role of the practical nurse in supporting the patient during the necessary changes is vital to success of any dietary modification. Any communication by the nurse, verbal or nonverbal, that indicates impatience, blame, or rejection of the patient for inability to accept the changes immediately or at the nurses' expected rate is inappropriate.

PROVIDING FOOD SERVICES FOR THE ELDERLY

The Need for Food Services

Many elderly couples and singles are able to live alone in safety. The security of living in surroundings that are familiar, whether it is a home, apartment, or a single room, is of great importance in maintaining independence. Food preparation and consumption is a key factor in the ability to keep this independence.

As physical and mental faculties are reduced, the task of food preparation may become insurmountable. Failing eyesight and shaky hands or loss of strength and energy may make working with stoves, knives, and appliances dangerous. Persons who are capable of these tasks may have temporary incapacities, such as broken limbs, surgery, or other problems. Some may be able to prepare the meal but unable to pay for food from almost nonexistent incomes. Single-room occupancy may not have provisions for food preparation. When the elderly are unable to care for their needs and there is no one to assist them, the only alternative may be placement in a nursing home.

Older persons who live alone often have no incentive to cook. They may eat carbohydrates to excess because they are easy to chew, require no preparation, and are inexpensive. (Robinson, Lawler, 1977, p. 333) Many elderly adults exist on tea and toast, dry cereals, or even pet foods. In our society, eating is usually a time when family members gather for sharing; being alone makes mealtime just another chore, easily neglected or skipped.

Operation of Food Services

In past chapters, we have discussed the dangers inherent in nursing-home placement. The cost for residency in a nursing home is great, both in terms of cost to society and trauma to the patient. The delivery of prepared food to the homes of the elderly on a regular or temporary basis will allow many people to retain their independence and stay at home longer.

"Meals on Wheels" or "Portable Meals" are meals that are usually prepared in a central place under directions available from the federal government for menu planning and nutritional content. The meals are delivered to the homes of the elderly once a day. While the programs vary in different regions, most of them deliver one hot meal and one smaller cold meal each day. Most programs are operated locally by volunteer groups such as churches, Golden Age clubs, and fraternal organizations. These are cost-sharing programs in most instances, and are designed particularly for those people who live alone. The cost to the elderly person is minimal or free, depending upon his circumstances. The demand for such food services outstrips the number in operation. Private concerns also offer food services, but their cost is prohibitive to many.

Delivery of meals to the homebound person is done by volunteers. This essential part of the service has proven to be of tremendous value. In many instances, the delivery person may be the only personal contact the elderly person has all day—or all week—with the outside world. Volunteers may be the first to learn of the elderly adult's other needs or illness and can summon help as necessary. The value of having someone to talk to is a great comfort and morale booster for the elderly person.

Other common programs are those meals served at midday in public schools or other public buildings. Congregate or communal meals are similar to school-lunch programs. Congregate meals, as well as the mobile programs, use standards formulated under the 1972 Federal Nutrition Plan for the Elderly. Menus for both use the four food groups and contain a higher nutrient density than other menus, although caloric totals are somewhat reduced. The reason for this is that the elderly require fewer calories, their basal metabolic rate is lower, and there is reduction of body size as well as a lower activity rate.

More recently, some nationwide chains of cafeterias have offered one or more meals per day at reduced costs to the elderly. These meals may be especially appealing, as they offer a variety of choices of food as well as the opportunity to see new faces and surroundings.

FOOD SERVICE IN THE NURSING HOME

The Dietary Department

The food-service division of any long-term care facility is an extremely important part of patient care. Diet can either provide a source of satisfaction or unhappiness and frustration to the patients.

The dietary department provides tray and dining-room service for residents of the nursing home. Unless the home is very large, the department is not staffed by a registered dietitian. The director of dietary services, who has taken a state-approved course in food management, is responsible for food service and kitchen personnel. A dietary consultant, who is a registered dietitian, visits periodically and assists with menus and checks the therapeutic diets and any other problems that may arise in skilled nursing homes.

Diet manuals, which list all of the diets served in the facility, should be available in the kitchen areas and at each nurses' station, so physicians and nurses have a ready reference.

Menus are made for one week for all diets and are recycled at about five-week intervals. This assures the patients of variety and assists the food department in planning and ordering supplies.

Sanitation and food storage regulations are imperative to assure a safe, clean food supply. All food handlers must have a current state food handler's permit to further protect the patient. Ideally, the person in charge of food service should visit each new resident and interview the person for knowledge of his usual food habits, likes and dislikes. The nursing personnel are responsible for carefully weighing and measuring of patients and noting if the patient is above or below his ideal body weight. These results should be noted on the patient's record and shared with the physician to assist him in ordering the most appropriate diet.

Some persons are admitted to long-term care facilities because they are unable to prepare their food or for other nutritionally related problems. These placements do not always guarantee that their nutritional level will be improved. Some studies (Tobias, 1977, p. 253–257; Brown, 1977, p. 41–45) show that patients in hospitals and nursing homes do not receive adequate balanced diets and that the caloric level may be just enough to meet metabolic requirements but insufficient for energy. Federal and state agencies monitor food service departments, but this does not assure compliance on a constant level.

Food-service departments of most long-term facilities offer many special services that are real morale builders. Each month, residents' birthdays are celebrated with a traditional cake and party. Holidays are occasions for special foods and many provide guest service for visiting relatives. Coffee and tea are made available most of the day for casual companionship.

There is always danger that mass-produced food can become tasteless and unattractive. The sight of a meal can mean as much to appetites as taste; it should be colorful and include a variety of consistencies. Many people feel that older adults prefer bland food and prepare food with this idea in mind. While highly spiced foods may be difficult to digest, the use of herbs, spices, lemon juice, or wine is essential to taste, particularly if the diet has sodium restrictions. Taste buds in elderly people have begun to decline in number; therefore foods need to be tasty for them to appreciate the flavors.

The food-service department may serve specific ethnic foods occasionally, according to the areas in which they are located. In Louisiana, it may be Cajun dishes; in Arizona, Mexican food; in the south, "soul" food. These dishes are usually looked forward to eagerly.

The preparation and serving of food in a long-term care facility is very important, not only from a dietary standpoint, but because mealtime may be the high point of the resident's day. A common observation is that of elderly men and women gathering together in the dining room an hour or more before serving time, as this is the most enjoyable time of the day. Socialization is easier, and sharing food and conversation seems a more normal activity than any other.

Facilities should have enough dining-room area to seat all of their residents. Eating with other people not only results in more satisfactory intake of food, but also keeps people in social contact with one another and assists in reality orientation of the individual. Every effort should be made to get all patients out of their rooms and into the dining room for meals. Patients who have hemiplegia, multiple sclerosis, arthritis, Parkinsonism, or who are blind may need special eating utensils. Many have learned to cope with the usual cutlery, but the nurse should be alert for special needs.

Those patients who go to the dining room for their meals are usually ambulatory and can tend to their own activities of daily living. Some patients who use wheelchairs may need assistance. It is important that they be able to arrive in the dining room at the correct time.

PREPARING BEDFAST PATIENTS FOR MEALS

When the food cart from the kitchen arrives on the patient unit, the trays are checked against a master diet list to ascertain that the correct diet is being served. Trays should be complete and arranged in an orderly manner.

The person who is either confined to bed or eats at the bedside must have an atmosphere of cleanliness and order in which to enjoy his meal. Oral care and personal hygiene should be completed before the arrival of a food tray. Preparation of patients for meals should have priority over any other nursing task except medical emergencies.

Careful assessment of which patients need to be fed is important, because over-solicitousness may result in the patient's loss of ability to do for himself. If the patient needs assistance or must be fed, this should be done immediately after the tray is delivered so food is hot when served. Feeding patients is not usually a favorite task of nursing personnel. If the nurse understands the meaning and importance of nutrition, she may be more patient and interested in the elderly adult's food intake. She should be comfortable, seated, if possible, while offering the food. Patients should always be in an upright position if at all possible. Placing the tray on an overbed table is advisable, rather than placing it on a bedside table. The sight and odor of food acts as an appetite stimulant.

The patient needs constant encouragement to participate in his feeding. Having the patient hold hand foods such as bread, bacon, or raw vegetables is a good way to start. In many instances, it is easier and quicker to feed a patient than to have him feed himself. This is a decided disservice, as it reduces his independence. Sometimes families wish to show their love and affection by feeding the patient when it is not really necessary. Careful explanations of why the patient must be involved in his own care can be helpful in assuring the family's support.

Tube Feeding

Some patients cannot be fed with a spoon because of their state of consciousness, or they may have some defect in the mouth. These patients can be successfully fed with a rubber-tipped syringe. Extreme care must be taken not to gag the patient and to proceed slowly so the patient does not become fatigued.

Other patients, who either (1) have difficulty or cannot swallow; (2) are unconscious or semiconscious; (3) cannot take enough food to maintain their bodies' demands; or (4) have difficulties retaining food, can be fed by gavage.

Gavage, or tube feedings, can be done by inserting a nasogastric tube into the stomach. A tube can also be inserted surgically into the esophagus (esophagostomy), into the stomach (gastrostomy), or jejunum (jejunostomy). The surgical procedures are done by the physician.

In any of the above methods, a liquid formula is used, composed of adequate carbohydrates, fats, and proteins. The physician prescribes the type, amount, and frequency of feedings. Sufficient fluids and medications can also be given through the tube. Commercial formulas are available, although the diet kitchen can provide a blenderized diet more economically.

The nurse should be very familiar with the facility's procedure for tube feedings before she attempts to give a formula. The procedure is not difficult, but there are specific precautions necessary to prevent aspiration and regurgitation of formula, as follows:

1. Only the amount and type of formula specified by the physician's orders should be given.

2. The specific amount of formula ordered is placed in a calibrated container, which is placed in warm, not hot, water. Hot water may cook the protein.

3. Elevate the bed to a sitting position, or place the patient on the right side with the head slightly elevated. When a tube is in the stomach, the cardiac sphincter that guards the esophageal opening into the stomach is kept open and will allow reflex action. The stomach contents can come back up the esophagus and be aspirated. Elevating the head prevents the back flow.

4. Adjust the flow of the formula. Approximately 30–45 minutes should be used for 200–300 milliliters of solution. Rapid

flow of the formula may result in diarrhea or regurgitation. If the rate is too slow, the prescribed amount of formula may be difficult to finish in a 24-hour period.

In some areas the initial tube placement is not done by the Practical Nurse, although she may be responsible for its maintenance. Formulas must be kept refrigerated until just before use. Holding the feeding at room temperature for any length of time encourages multiplication of bacteria.

Preparation of the patient for the feeding, as well as oral care and nasal care, are as important as for any patient before any meal.

Charting following the feedings should indicate the amount and type of feeding as well as the amount of fluid given prior to and after the feeding. The patient's reaction to the feeding is also important.

NUTRITIONAL PROBLEMS IN CHRONIC CONDITIONS

Special Diets

The older person who can eat all foods and whose health is good is fortunate. The elderly have many chronic conditions that may indicate the need for a special diet. Therapeutic diets are modifications of the normal nutritional requirements developed to meet the needs of the body with specific diseases.

Oral Problems

The assimilation of all diets, whether normal or therapeutic, is affected by the condition of the patient's teeth. All teeth may be missing, or dentures may be poorly fitted. If dentures are to fit correctly, the health of the gums is very important. If dentures are unusable or absent, all food may have to be ground in order to facilitate chewing. Such a diet is called a Mechanical Soft Diet.

The use of ground meats or pureed foods is not well accepted by most people. The original appearance of the food is totally destroyed. A great percentage of our appetite is stimulated by the enjoyment we feel at seeing colorful, well prepared food. In many instances the food-service department serves pureed foods in several bowls without setting up a regular tray. This further destroys the normalcy of the person's meal. Nursing personnel are also affected by the sight, and many report they dislike feeding ground and pureed foods. If meats are minced finely, rather than ground, they retain much of their original character. Although minced meats may be difficult to chew, most people prefer them to ground consistencies. Even edentulous patients can manage quite well with some assistance. Care should be taken that food is in small enough bites so that choking is prevented. Ideally, the patient should be fitted with dentures, but this is not always possible.

Diet in Chronic Disease Conditions

Chronic conditions increase with age and cause increasing disability. The most common conditions that require dietary intervention are cardiac, diabetic, and hypertension problems. The goals of cardiac dietary plans are (1) maximum rest for the heart; (2) prevention or elimination of edema; (3) maintenance of good nutrition; and (4) acceptability of the program by the patient. (Robinson and Lawler, 1977, p. 541) Three common restrictions in diets are usually prescribed for cardiac problems; they are:

1. Fat-controlled diets for atherosclerosis
2. Sodium-restricted diets for retention of fluids
3. Weight reduction for hypertension.

Fat-controlled diets for atherosclerosis

Fat consumption in the United States is approximately 100 pounds per person. This can be safely reduced by 35 percent. (Williams, 1974, p. 251)

Atherosclerosis is a pathological condition of the major blood vessels. Thickening of the vessels by fatty plaques reduces the size of the lumen. This narrowing results in less blood flow and the increased possibility of blood clots in the vessel. The absence of nutrients and oxygen to cells results in death or infarct of the tissue. When this occurs in heart muscle, myocardial infarct or heart attack results.

Atherosclerosis can be controlled by reducing animal fat and using vegetable sources of fat. Specific diet lists can be obtained from the American Heart Association.

Sodium restriction for retention of fluids

In congestive heart failure, the heart is no longer able to maintain its normal blood circulation. The result is retention of fluid throughout the body, including the pleural cavity. Respirations become difficult, and the additional fluids cause the weakened heart additional labor. Hormonal imbalance in congestive heart failure results in increased fluid retention. The goals of edema control are to reduce the sodium intake as little as possible, but enough to result in diuresis. Once edema has been satisfactorily reduced, moderate restriction (1,000 mg.) may be all that is required, if any.

In long-term facilities, diets are provided for sodium restriction from 1,000 mg. (1 gm) to 4,500 mg. (4.5 gm) of sodium. Patients with diets that require less than 1 gm. of sodium are usually candidates for transfer to an acute care facility.

Table 8-2 shows an example of a form for ordering a patient's diet. This form encourages the physician to order specific diets to conform to the dietary modifications used in the facility. The specific order from the doctor reduces confusion and assures the right diet for the patient.

Low-sodium diets are rather tasteless, and their degree of appeal depends in large measure on the amount of salt the individual has

TABLE 8-2

ORDER FORM FOR SODIUM-RESTRICTED DIET
Patient's name _____ Room # _____
DOCTOR: Please check which sodium restricted diet you are prescribing for your patient.
Sodium restriction—moderate   1000 mg.   _____ Sodium restriction-mild   2000 mg. to 4500   _____ Remove extra salt from tray only   _____
(Date)   Physician's signature

A complete list of food restrictions are available in the diet manual at each chart desk. For questions, dial Dietary Service at Ext. 498.

used in the past. The patient must fully understand the reason for the restriction and receive support to adhere to the diet. The use of various spices, herbs, citrus juices, and physician-approved salt substitutes can result in meals as appetizing as any other. A sodium-restricted diet plus medication usually results in dramatic improvement of the edema, which results in less difficult respirations. These results may assist in motivating the patient to accept the diet. The nurse must check food trays to be sure of the correct diet, with no additional salt provided. Specific detailed diet information is available from the American Heart Association.

Patients with chronic cardiac problems, hypertension, and other health problems may have diuretic medications prescribed to reduce the total circulating fluid in the body, which reduces the work load of the heart. In diuresis, fluid readsorption from the renal tubules is reduced, and potassium is lost through the urine. Potassium is also lost if diarrhea and vomiting occur. Normal potassium levels (3.8 to 5.0 mEq./L) are essential to the maintenance of normal sodium balance (136 to 142 mEq./L.) and normal acid-base balance (7.38 to 7.44 whole arterial blood, 7.36 to 7.41 whole venous blood).

Following episodes of diarrhea, vomiting, and diuretic intake, the body needs potassium replacement by use of high potassium foods such as meat, poultry, fish, nuts, spinach, whole grain cereals, legumes, milk solids, and fruits such as tomatoes, citrus, prunes and bananas. Tea, coffee, and chocolate or cocoa drinks also contain potassium, but may be contraindicated because of other physical factors.

Hypertension

Hypertension can be defined as blood pressure elevated above 150 systolic and 90 diastolic that remains at that level over a period of time. Hypertension is a complex of symptoms, often present in cardiovascular and renal diseases. Essential hypertension (cause unknown) is the most common, 80 to 90 percent of the people with high blood pressure are in this category.

Increased blood pressure may occur with no apparent symptoms. If symptoms do appear, the patient may complain of fatigue, headache, or apprehension. If there is a cardiac problem, dyspnea, palpitations, and retention of fluid may also occur. Attacks of vertigo and fainting may also be experienced.

If the patient is overweight, reduction of weight may be enough to lower the blood pressure. Sodium restriction will also cause temporary weight reduction, even though it may be temporary. A variety of antihypertensive drugs are available to the physician.

When the patient begins to recover from acute cardiac problems or when his blood pressure is reduced and he feels well, the need for long-term dietary care and medications may seem unimportant. Constant encouragement and reinforcement of teaching is necessary to help the patient remain on his medication and diet routine.

The diabetic diet

The elderly adult who is a diabetic at present probably has the maturity-onset form of the disease. Insulin, discovered in 1922, was the first treatment other than diet control. Therefore, persons with the juvenile-onset form of diabetes who had insulin treatment and survived would rarely be found in institutions because their total numbers would be small.

Maturity onset diabetes develops slowly. Its symptoms are milder than juvenile onset, and the patient's condition is more stable. The danger of acidosis is not as great, and the disease can usually be controlled by diet restrictions. If additional control is necessary, oral hypoglycemic agents can be used and are effective in about 40 percent of the cases. Insulin is necessary in about 20–30 percent of the mature-onset diabetics.

Diet is the most important treatment for the diabetic person. Carbohydrate, fat, and protein intake must be controlled. Exercise and medications are balanced with diet to avoid the complications of diabetic coma, insulin shock, hypoglycemia, and hyperglycemia.

The changes in diet necessary for the diabetic patient are as difficult for him as for any other patient who must change his patterns of eating.

The goals for the diabetic diet are as follows:

1. To correct weight to the individual's ideal weight and maintain it at that level.
2. To maintain a good nutritional level.
3. To maintain control of the disease.

The diet will be prescribed by the physician, who orders specific percentages of carbohydrates, fat, and protein. The American Diabetic

Association recommends 50-60 percent carbohydrate, 10-15 percent protein, and 30-35 percent fat. Some physicians prefer a 40-20-40 formula because the high carbohydrate percentage of the ADA diet is not always well tolerated.

One of the greatest problems for the elderly adult in adhering to the dietary changes is in convincing himself he really needs to change. Because the disease is not as severe as the juvenile type, he may feel better with the use of hypoglycemic medications. After some dietary indiscretion, he may notice no particular adverse symptoms. This persuades him that he is not really in need of change.

The practical nurse and the dietitian must continue to emphasize the need for diet and the need to avoid the complications possible when the disease is not controlled.

It is probably easier for the adult in the nursing home to comply with his diet, as he does not have to plan and prepare the meal. It is always possible to deviate from the plan regardless of where one is, and the patient should not be made to feel guilty when this occurs. It should also be emphasized that failing to eat the diet prepared is just as dangerous as eating additional foods.

Nurses should be alert, particularly between meals, for hypoglycemic reactions. These occur with the patients taking oral medication as well as those on insulin.

Oral hypoglycemics should never be given at night, as the long period without food intake can result in low blood sugar during that time. Any symptom such as irritability, nervousness, dizziness, lethargy, headache, sweating, hunger, shakiness, tremors, or palpitations indicate hypoglycemia. These symptoms may not be caused by overdosage of the hypoglycemic medication, but by taking it at the wrong time. Fruit juice, soft drinks, candy, or other high carbohydrate foods will combat the symptoms.

The patient taking insulin who has not eaten his meal, or who has exercised beyond his normal limits, may also experience hypoglycemia and have the same symptoms as listed above.

Constant observation of the diabetics' diet and other precautions to avoid complications are necessary to safeguard these patients.

REVIEW QUESTIONS

1. Why are changes in diet difficult to maintain?
2. Why is it necessary to have sufficient carbohydrates in the diet?

3. List at least four problems that might face the elderly person who is trying to provide himself an adequate diet.

4. Give three reasons for caloric reduction in the diet of the elderly adult.

5. Of what importance is limitation of sodium in the cardiac diet?

6. What type of diet would be indicated for the person with atherosclerosis?

7. If a patient must be fed, what actions of the nurse will help assure that the patient has a pleasant mealtime?

RECOMMENDED ACTIVITIES

1. Plan a balanced meal for one week for an elderly person at the lowest cost possible. Compare in class and discuss the methods for saving you used.

2. Interview a person who delivers "Meals on Wheels." What does the person feel she gains from such a voluntary service? If such a program is not available in your area, interview any volunteer who works with the elderly.

3. Interview an elderly person who is independent. Does this person have any problems with diet? Preparation of food? Cost? Is he on a therapeutic diet? What strengths did the person show in maintaining his independence?

BIBLIOGRAPHY

Brown, Phyllis et al. "Dietary Status of Elderly People." *Journal American Diabetic Association* 70 (January 1977): 15-19.

Chaney, Patricia S., ed. *Managing Diabetics Properly*. Horsham, Penn.: Intermed Communications, Inc. Nursing 77 Skillbook Series, 1977, Chapter 3.

Evans, Richard, and Yolanda Hall. "Social-Psychologic Perceptives of Motivating Changes in Eating Behavior." *Journal of the American Dietetic Association* 72 (April 1978): 378-382.

Harper, J.M. et al. "Menu Planning in the Nutrition Program for the Elderly." *Journal of the American Dietetic Association* 68 (June 1976): 529-534.

Robinson, Corrine, and Marilyn R. Lawler. *Normal and Therapeutic Nutrition*, 15th ed. New York: Macmillan, 1977.

Tobias, Alice L., and Theodore B. Van Itallie. "Nutritional Problems of Hospitalized Patients." *Journal of the American Dietetic Association* 71 (September 1977): 253-257.

United States Department of Health, Education and Welfare. *Facts on Older Americans*. Washington, D.C., 1973.

United States Department of Agriculture. *Toward the New*. Washington, D.C.: Bulletin 341, 1972.

Wainwright, Helen. "Feeding Problems in Elderly Disabled Patients." *Nursing Times* 74 (March 30, 1978): 542-543.

Weber, Helen I. "Continuity of Care." Speech, A.N.A. Workshop: Care of the Elderly, Phoenix, Arizona, 1972.

Williams, Sue Rodwell. *Essentials of Nutrition and Diet Therapy*. St. Louis: C.V. Mosby Co., 1974.

Young, C.M. "Interviewing the Patient." *American Journal of Clinical Nutrition* 8 (August 1960): 523.

chapter 9

Problems Concerned with Emergency Situations in the Elderly

OBJECTIVES

After studying this unit, the student will be able to:

1. Describe why early detection of changes in the elderly is important.

2. Explain why philosophies of care differ in acute care and long-term care facilities.

3. Discuss the value of taking frequent vital signs in the care facilities.

4. List some indicators of impending illness other than abnormal vital signs in the elderly.

5. Describe how you would know that behavioral changes were not caused by normal mental deterioration.

Emergency situations in the care of the elderly person are similar to those found in other age groups. Myocardial infarction, cerebral vascular accidents, and traumatic injuries all occur in long-term care facilities. The heroic measures utilized in hospitals have no place in the care of the elderly patient in a nursing home. He does deserve good nursing care, which incorporates preventative care and rapid, accurate assessment of signs and symptoms that may indicate new problems that, if treated, can restore the patient to his former level of health.

The philosophy of care given to the elderly adult in a long-term care facility is different from the care in an acute care center. In the acute center, the aim is to cure and/or improve the patient's condition. In long-term care, the most important goal is to maintain independence of mind and body, to protect the patient, and to allow the patient to die with dignity.

One of the hazards of old age is a predisposition to certain diseases, and most people die of these diseases rather than of old age. Cardiovascular and respiratory diseases and cancer are well-known common killers of the aged. The susceptibility to them and to other diseases results from the patient's inability to maintain homeostasis.

IMPORTANCE OF EARLY ASSESSMENT OF ILLNESS

The balance between illness and health in the elderly is precarious. Normal aging results in a decrease of functional capabilities and a decrease in the function of synchronizing systems of the body. The changes in the immune system of the body are among the most important, as the antibodies' ability to react to new antigens is so reduced that infections become more common. The reserves of strength

187

and energy are reduced, and the person is more susceptible to disease. If the patient becomes ill, death is more likely than in former years, regardless of the cause. Recovery from illness or trauma is slower, and complications are more common and severe.

The delicate balance of the health of the elderly makes it important to detect any changes in the patient, whether physical or mental, before a disease condition progresses.

OBSERVING FOR IMPORTANT PHYSICAL AND BEHAVIORAL CHANGES

There are no new measurements of body functions in the care of the elderly. The same procedures are carried out with the same tools, and the same observations are made as with any other group of patients. Nurses develop the ability to learn about patients by listening to them and studying their actions and appearance and taking their measurements. The difference lies in the interpretation of the data that is collected. Interpretation cannot be logical unless the data gathered is accurate and complete. The norms usually accepted are somewhat altered in the older adult.

The Vital Signs

Many long-term care facilities do not take vital signs more than once a month, usually just prior to developing a report for the doctor when he renews medication orders. The patients who have been judged most acutely ill may have their vital signs taken frequently, but the value of infrequent measurements on other patients who may have a number of chronic diseases is negligible.

The facility's patient-care committee may set guidelines for more frequent measurement of vital signs. The charge nurse, however, who knows the diagnoses and conditions of the patients on her unit, may order them taken as she feels necessary for certain specific patients. Frequent measurements are necessary so that an accurate data base of information about the patient is available for comparison of future measurement. In this way, a norm can be established for each patient who is an individual with variations from the general norm.

Temperatures that are above 99.5° F (37.5° C) orally, or 100.5° F (38.0° C) rectally, are commonly considered elevated. The elderly adult, however, due to normal deterioration of the central nervous system, may not have a temperature elevated to that which we accept as abnormal. Therefore, a baseline temperature, taken at different times of the day, is essential in judging whether the patient has a fever.

The method by which the temperature is taken must be evaluated by the nurse. The oral thermometer should be in place at least 8-9 minutes. While this route is the most acceptable to patients, mouth breathers, those using oxygen equipment, or comotose or confused patients should have rectal temperatures taken. Rectal thermometers should be in place at least 3 minutes. If the patient is confused or agitated, the rectal temperature may prove to further upset the patient, and so axillary temparatures may need to be considered. The thermometer should be in place ten minutes.

In addition to the measurement of temperature with a thermometer, the nurse should also observe other signs that indicate there is an abnormal temperature disturbance. Observation of the skin may result in such findings as "skin cold, clammy, hot, dry, or reddened." The patient may be shivering or complaining of a chill. Skin that is dry, with dry mucous membrane, indicates dehydration with elevated temperature.

The cardiac output and the stroke volume of the heart in elderly adult patients is decreased. Therefore, the pulse rate increases to assure a constant cardiac output. The pulse, usually taken at the radial artery, may be taken apically with the use of the stethescope.

The elderly adult's pulse may range from 60-100 or slightly higher. When counting the pulse, the rhythm, force, and quality are also noted. If there are irregularities, the pulse deficit should be noted. The difference between radial and apical pulse taken simultaneously by two persons is the deficit, and should be reported to the charge nurse and physician. The deficit results from two beats of the heart that come very close together. The second beat pumps little blood from the heart, as the left ventricle does not have enough time between beats to fill with blood. The greater the rate of the deficit, the more serious the disturbance of the heart beat, or arrhythmia.

Respiratory rates also change, as maximum oxygen uptake and vital capacity is reduced. These changes may be caused by pulmonary disease, such as emphysema, bronchiectasis, or even poor posture. Cardiac efficiency and the oxygen transport system may also cause the respiratory rate to decrease. The normal rate of respiration in adults is 18 per minute, and is the count of the rhythmic rising and falling of the chest wall. Respiration is normally counted with the fingers still on the pulse to reduce anxiety. Normally the ratio of respiration to pulse is about 1:4 or 1:5, but in disease states both increase. In respiratory problems, the pulse increases, but the respirations increase much more, and the ratio may be nearer 1:9 or 1:10. While taking the pulse, the nurse should observe how the patient positions himself. Does he need to sit up, do respirations seem labored or painful? The movements of the chest and abdomen are also noted. What is the color of the patient's face, lips, fingernails, and ear lobes?

Blood-pressure readings for the elderly were once felt to be normally higher than those for the younger age groups. The popular slogan "one hundred plus your age" was accepted. Threshold levels

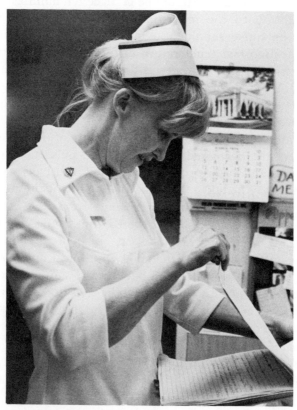

Photographer: Doris Wilson, RN
Model: Ava Mills

The practical nurse reviews the data base to evaluate new information about the patient's condition.

for persons over 50 at present indicate that diastolic pressure of 90 mm Hg. or above requires further monitoring. When 95 mm Hg. are reached, treatment is indicated. Systolic pressure of 150 mm Hg. is considered for further monitoring, while a resting pressure of over 160 mm Hg. is hypertensive.

If the nursing personnel are not aware of the normal variance of vital signs in the elderly, they cannot make accurate judgments concerning the need for further monitoring or reporting the patient's condition to the charge nurse or physician.

A common practice on nursing units is to have one person take vital signs on all the patients. If all nursing personnel are qualified to take vital signs, it is better nursing practice for the person caring for the patient to take the vital signs. Slight fluctuations may seem meaningless to some nurses, while the one most knowledgeable concerning the patient may pick up other clues.

Taking vital signs is one of the earliest nursing techniques learned. Once the procedure is mastered, it appears simple, and its value may not be understood by personnel. The licensed practical nurse must be alert to the danger of using less than precise techniques in her practice. She must also, cooperating with the registered nurse, assure herself of the accuracy of the techniques of the nursing assistants who may be her responsibility. If there is any doubt, vital signs must be rechecked for accuracy. Reteaching to prevent repetitive checking, which is unpleasant and anxiety producing for the patient, may also be indicated.

Other Indicators

Another sign that may alert the nurse to a patient's illness is loss of appetite. If the patient has tray service in the room, a lagging appetite is easy to detect. It does require a careful check of each tray as it is removed from the room, and an immediate notation of the amount of food consumed. If the nature of the appetite is not recorded promptly, serious malnutrition and weight loss can occur before it becomes apparent.

Many patients have their meals in the dining room, and if there are no nursing personnel assigned to the area, knowledge of anorexia may be delayed.

If the patient has been eating poorly, checking for the reason may result in finding that the patient has painful ulcerations on the lips or in the mouth, or swallowing may be difficult. Failure to eat may also be a covert suicide attempt.

Elderly persons can lose weight rapidly, resulting in loss of strength, fatigue, and loss of resistance. Admission weight and at least monthly checks are indicated for an accurate data base. The use of bed scales for those unable to stand seems essential, as these patients may need the most accurate monitoring.

A sudden change in the level of activity is also significant in the assessment of the elderly patient's health. The patient who is normally up and about may suddenly not want to get out of bed, or he may doze in a chair all day.

Situations of grave concern in caring for the elderly may not be considered emergencies in younger age groups. The delicate balance of homeostasis in the older group makes quick detection and treatment imperative to the life of the elderly adult.

Common Emergencies

Most emergency situations that occur in caring for the elderly result from complications or exacerbations of diseases already present, except for traumatic injuries. Infections are one of the most frequently occurring problems that can be difficult to detect if nurses are not constantly vigilant for obscure clues.

Infections

Respiratory infections are among the most common problems of the elderly. Hypostatic pneumonia is particularly common when the patient has been immobilized for some time.

Aspiration pneumonia in the comatose or weak patient may result from the inability to cough up secretions from the throat and bronchi. Improperly managed tube feedings may also cause aspiration.

Lobar pneumonia, commonly caused by staphylococcus, Friedlander's bacillus, or Hemophilus influenzae, and atypical (viral) pneumonia are also prevalent.

Confusion, malaise, cough, dyspnea, and increased temperature are typical symptoms of respiratory infections. Profuse diaphoresis, common in pneumonia, may be absent. The elderly may not exhibit these common symptoms, and only persistent cough and malaise may occur.

The mortality rate in respiratory infections is high in the elderly, and detection must occur quickly for diagnostic procedures and treatment to begin.

Influenza, which seems to occur in cycles, is also a dangerous problem for the elderly because of the changes in the cardiopulmonary system. Communal living increases the exposure of the patients when one is ill. The best treatment, therefore, is prevention. The Center for Disease Control in Atlanta, Georgia, recommends that all persons 65 years and older, and all who have debilitating diseases, receive an annual flu vaccination.

Because of the slowness with which the elderly's body defense mechanisms respond to the invasion of infectious organisms, the disease may be well developed before there is an increase of temperature and leukocytosis. The patient may even die before such indicators are evident. The same condition in a younger patient would be evident much sooner, and could be treated vigorously with satisfactory prognosis.

Urinary tract infections are quite prevalent, particularly cystitis in the elderly female. These infections are usually insidious in their onset. The cause of the infection may be urinary retention of residual urine, obstructions in the urinary tract and the use of indwelling catheters. The causative organisms commonly found are *Escherichia coli, Streptococcus,* and *Proteus.*

The usual symptoms of frequency, urgency, and pain or burning upon voiding and hematuria that indicate urinary-tract infections may be missing. The subtle changes that were discussed previously may be the only indications of the infection, and urinalysis and urine culture are indicated when there is any suspicion.

The elderly male may have general malaise caused by urinary tract infection, with retention of urine. Frequency of urination in small amounts and nocturia with eventual retention give the clues to this problem. In many instances, benign prostatic hypertrophy may be the cause, and surgery will be indicated.

Not only are beginning infections difficult to detect, but other serious diseases such as myocardial infarcts, mild cerebral vascular accidents, and others have diminished symptoms at times. This makes knowledge of the patient, good baseline data, and accurate measurement of vital signs with careful study of laboratory reports vital to giving the best of care to the elderly adult.

Not all elderly persons have diminution of symptoms. Some will present the same picture of vital signs that other age groups do. It is just as important to know which patients have these patterns as to detect the more elusive symptoms of others.

Behavioral Changes

Physical and behavioral observations are divided here for clarity. In reality, these observations occur simultaneously, and are part of the whole person.

A change in behavior may be the only overt sign of a physical or mental change in the patient, and merits further investigation. Behavioral changes must be evaluated by asking the following: (1) Is this behavior part of the patient's normal personality? Harry Jones has always walked rapidly up and down halls swinging his arms in circles every fifth step because ten years ago a doctor told him it helped circulation. (2) Could the behavior be due to medication? Lisa Adams, usually alert and able to move easily, sits in an armchair, slumped over with hand dragging on the floor, and does not respond well to questions. Yesterday, her usual mild tranquilizer was changed to a new product. (3) What other nonphysical causes could explain the behavior? Lola Grimes goes from door to door looking in at each room, finally enters a vacant one and lies down on the bed. Last evening Mrs. Grimes was moved to a new room when the thermostat failed to function. (4) What physical reason might cause the behavioral change? Nellie Smithers is lying in bed moaning and refuses to get up as she usually does. Upon questioning her, she states she fell in the bathroom last night, and has a large hematoma on her hip and thigh.

When no apparent reasons for the change in behavior can be found, then careful measurement of vital signs must be done in an attempt to detect whether physical and mental changes seem indicative of more serious problems. Some of the common behavioral changes are agitation, confusion, disorientation, mental dullness, and loss of memory.

Nonverbal clues may also help detect problems. Facial expressions may help to detect pain, disorientation, and fear. The body may be held in such a manner that fatigue, pain, and tremors may be evident.

REPORTING AND RECORDING CHANGES

When a complete assessment of vital signs, observations, and interview of the patient with comparison of past data, and laboratory reports have been made, and the results indicate that there is a possibility that the patient is experiencing physical or mental problems, the physician should be contacted for a report on the change in the patient's condition.

In reporting to the doctor, the following points should be kept in mind:

1. It may be several months since the doctor last saw his patient, so he needs to be updated.

"Mrs. Effie Morris is an 86-year-old who was admitted January 15, 1979. Her admitting diagnosis was diabetes mellitus and osteogenic arthritis. She is currently on regular Insulin 20U q.d., 1500 Cal. Diabetic Diet, and Aspirin grains 10 tid. Since yesterday, she has been lethargic, had a poor appetite, and been very irritable. Her clinitest is 1+, and acetone is negative. Her vital signs are normal for her: T-98 P-108 R-22. She says she has no pain. Her urine, however, is very concentrated and has a foul odor. We have been encouraging fluids."

This type of report refreshes the doctor's memory of the patient, states the signs and symptoms, and tells him what, if anything, has been done for the patient.

2. In an emergency situation, give only the most obvious facts— you need help fast.

"Doctor, your patient, Mrs. Fox, has fallen in her bathroom. There is a one-inch laceration in the left frontal region; pressure has been applied. The left femur is out of alignment midway between hip and knee; the skin is not broken. She has been covered, left in the position where she fell; she is conscious and oriented. The pupils are equal and react to light. She is very anxious but does not seem to be in severe pain. Pulse is 110—blood pressure 158/90. The ambulance has been called; they know there is a possible fracture.

This rapid report informs the doctor what has happened, that there is no apparent brain injury, and that the fracture is not compound. The ambulance attendants will be prepared to splint the leg before moving. You are basically asking for permission to transport the patient and awaiting his orders.

3. In reporting, the following facts should also be collected before the physician is contacted:

A. Complete vital signs, with a statement comparing them to past measurements. In emergency situations, the signs most pertinent to the patient's condition are the essential ones.

B. A description of the patient's subjective symptoms—how the patient describes his problem.

C. What the nurse observes, the patient's objective symptoms. These may be a redness of skin, rash, shivering, or other abnormal conditions.

Reports such as these will assist the physician in changing or discontinuing old orders, ordering new treatments or medications, ordering diagnostic testing, or deciding that he needs to see the patient or to have him transferred for acute care.

In addition to relaying these facts to the doctor, the practical nurse shares her findings with the charge nurse or with a supervisor. They are also entered into the patient's record with a further notation that the supervisor, head nurse, and doctor were notified.

Accurate assessment and reporting, both verbal and written, are essential parts of comprehensive care of the elderly adult.

REVIEW QUESTIONS

1. Why do respiratory rates and pulse rates usually increase in the elderly?

2. If you find the patient's blood pressure is 165/100 upon admission, what would you do?
3. Why is it difficult for the elderly adult to maintain homeostasis?
4. Explain why it is important to establish and maintain a data base of the patient's vital signs and weight.
5. Explain why the elderly adult can have an infection and still have normal vital signs.

BIBLIOGRAPHY

Beletz, Elaine E., and Gabriela A. Covo. "The Case of the Hidden Infections in the Elderly." *Nursing '76* 6 (August 1976): 14–16.

_____ *Assessing Vital Functions Accurately.* Horsham, Pennsylvania: Intermed Communications, Inc., 1977.

Butler, Robert N., and Myrna Lewis. *Aging and Mental Health.* St. Louis: C.V. Mosby Company, 1977.

Falconer, Mary W. et al. *Aging Patients; a Guide for Their Care.* New York: Springer Publishing Co., 1976.

Hasler, Doris. *The Practical Vocational Nurse and Today's Family,* 2d ed. New York: Macmillan, 1972.

Henderson, Virginia, and Gladys Hite. *Principles and Practice of Nursing,* 6th ed. New York: Macmillan, 1978, Chapters 6, 8.

Jaeger, Dorothea, and Leo W. Simmons. *The Aged Ill.* New York: Appleton-Century-Crofts, 1970.

Nichols, Glennadee A., and Dolores H. Kucha. "Taking Adult Temperatures: Oral Measurement." *American Journal of Nursing* 72 (June, 1972): 1091.

Glossary

accountability   the nurse's responsibility to be answerable, to define, or explain her actions.

acidosis   a pathological condition, results from an accumulation of acid or loss of base from the body.

A.D.L.   activities of daily living, such as personal hygiene, dressing, toileting, feeding one's self, ability to move or walk.

Alzheimer's disease   a degenerative organic disease generally occurring in middle life.

amyloid placques   starchlike deposits in specific tissues.

antibody   a substance in the body that produces immunity (antagonistic to invading bodies) such as the reacting agents in serum.

anticoagulant   1. acting to prevent clotting of blood. 2. any substance that suppresses, delays, or nullifies blood coagulation.

antigen   any substance that is capable of producing antibody formation and reacting in a detectable way with the antibodies produced.

anorexia   loss or lack of appetite for food.

aspiration   the act of inhaling a fluid.

atherosclerosis   a form of arteriosclerosis in which fatty deposits are formed in large- and medium-sized arteries.

atrophy   a wasting away or reduction in size of a cell, tissue, organ, or part.

atypical   irregular, not conforming to type.

bacillus   a genus of bacteria including gram positive, spore forming bacteria.

behavior modification   a method of reeducation based upon Pavlovian conditioning. Behavior will change when change is rewarded.

Bennett respirator   a type of machine used for intermittent positive pressure breathing.

Bird respirator   a type of machine used for intermittent positive pressure breathing.

body image   the individual's perception of one's body, both consciously and unconsciously.

brain syndrome   1. **acute**, reversible impaired brain function. 2. **chronic**, irreversible impaired brain function. 3. **organic**, a group of symptoms resulting from impaired brain function. May be acute or chronic.

cachectic   a state of malnutrition, general illness and body wasting.

calibrated   divided, marked with graduations, as a thermometer, measuring cup.

carcinoma   a synonym for cancer.

cardiac sphincter   the muscle located at the cardiac portion of the stomach at the esophagogastric junction.

cerebro-vascular accident (stroke)   a condition with sudden onset caused by acute vascular lesions of the brain (hemorrhage, embolism, thrombosis, etc.) that may result in paralysis of one-half the body, slight paralysis of one side of the body, vertigo, numbness, loss of speech, difficulty in moving joints, and often permanent neurological damage.

charge nurse   the nurse responsible for a given number of patients and for the personnel management and other administrative duties of a specific area. Also known as head nurse, unit director, etc.

contractures abnormal shortening of muscle tissue, which makes the muscle resistant to stretching.

covert concealed or secret.

cupping lightly striking the upper body with hands held in a cupped position.

cyanosis slightly bluish, grayish, slatelike or dark purple discoloration of the skin.

day care a program in which elderly persons are cared for a certain number of hours a day, returning home at night.

dementia organic loss of intellectual function. 1. **arteriosclerotic d**, intellectual function loss due to arteriosclerotic changes in the brain. 2. **senile d.**, mental deterioration in old age, organic brain changes; symptoms include impaired memory for recent events, irritability, etc.

diabetes, juvenile onset a chronic systemic disease with disorders in the metabolism of insulin, carbohydrates, fats, and proteins. Usually occurs before age 20, but may be later.

diabetes, maturity onset chronic systemic disease with disorders in the metabolism of insulin, carbohydrates, fats, and proteins. Usually occurs after age 30, but may occur earlier.

diaphoreses profuse sweating.

diuretic any agent that increases urine output.

dyspnea labored or difficult breathing, may be accompanied by pain.

edema an abnormal accumulation of fluid in intercellular spaces of the body.

edentulous without teeth.

electrolyte a substance that dissociates into ions fused in solution, thus becoming capable of conducting electricity.

embolus a clot or other plug brought by the blood from another vessel and forced into a smaller one, which obstructs the circulation.

Escherichia coli the *Bacillus coli communis*, a colon bacterium, usually nonpathogenic.

esophagostomy a creation of an opening into the esophagus.

exacerbation   aggravation of symptoms or increase in the severity of a disease.

exudate   a fluid with a high protein content and dead cells that has escaped from blood vessels and is deposited in tissues or tissue surfaces as a result of inflammation.

gastrostomy   creation of an artificial opening in the stomach.

Gatch   the movable portion of a hospital bed that can be raised or lowered at the head or under knees.

gavage   feeding through a tube passed into the stomach.

geriatric   the care of the aged.

gerontology   the study of the problems of the aged in all its aspects.

gingiva   the mucous membrane, with supporting fibrous tissue, covering the toothbearing border of the jaw.

homemaker services   services that the person may be given such as personal care, care of the environment, food preparation, marketing, or specific health care.

homeostasis   a tendency to stability in the normal physiological states of the organism.

hyperglycemia   an excess of glucose in the blood.

hypertension   persistent high arterial blood pressure.

hypoglycemia   a deficiency of sugar in the blood, a condition that may lead to nervousness, hypothermia, headache, confusion, and sometimes convulsions and coma.

hypoglycemic agents   drugs that lower the glucose content of the blood, such as sulfonylureas and biguanides.

hypotension   abnormally low blood pressure.

hypothermia   the abnormal lowering of body temperature.

ilium, crest of   the upper margin of the hip bone.

immune   being highly resistant to a disease because of formation of antibodies.

incontinence   the inability to retain either urine or feces.

influenza   a viral infection of the respiratory tract, caused by types A, B, and C virus.

inhalation therapy   treatment that assists persons with respiratory problems, for example, oxygen administration, IPPF treatments.

inhalation therapy technician   a specially prepared person who gives inhalation therapy treatments.

institution   in this text used as a title for any building devoted primarily to the care of the elderly adult.

insulin   a protein hormone secreted by beta cells of the pancreas. Also a drug manufacturered mainly for the treatment of diabetes.

intermediate care   that designation by the Department of Health, Education and Welfare for Medicare patients in nursing homes who do not require 24-hour professional nursing care.

intermittent positive pressure breathing   forces increased inspiratory breathing. Also used to designate machines used in the treatment. Abbreviated IPPB.

jejunostomy   the creation of a permanent opening between the jejunum and the surface of the abdominal wall.

labium   pl. *labia*   the elongated fold on the sides of the vaginal orifice.

leukocytosis   an increase in the number of leukocytes (white blood cells) in the blood due to various causes.

long-term care facility   used synonymously with *institution, facility*, and *nursing home* to designate a place where the elderly are cared for under state and/or federal regulations. Indicates care necessary for thirty days or more.

macerated   tissue that has been softened by wetting or soaking.

maceration   process of softening a solid by steeping in fluid.

malaise   a vague feeling of bodily discomfort.

meatus, external urinary   the opening of the urethra on the body surface through which urine is discharged.

Medicaid   a government program financed by federal, state, and local funds, providing hospitalization and medical insurance for persons of all ages within certain income limits.

Medicare   a federal program of hospitalization insurance and voluntary medical insurance for persons aged 65 and over.

Medicare certification   that certification given to long-term care facilities that meet the requirements of DHEW and the individual states for standards of care.

mores   customs or folkways of importance, accepted by a certain segment of society.

multiple sclerosis   chronic induration in patches scattered over the nervous system.

neurofibril   one of the delicate threads running in every direction through the nerve cells.

neuropsychiatric   a combination of neurological and psychiatric problems.

nocturia   excessive urination at night.

necrotic   relating to death of a portion of tissue.

nosocomial   infections that originate in hospitals or other health care institutions.

nurse, licensed practical/vocational   a graduate of a school of practical/vocational nursing whose qualifications have been examined by the state board of nursing and who has been legally authorized to practice as a licensed practical or vocational nurse (LPN-LVN) under the supervision of a physician or registered nurse. **n. registered**   a graduate nurse who has been legally authorized (registered) to practice after examination by the state board of nurse examiners or similar regulatory authority, and who is legally entitled to use the designation R.N.

nursing home   a facility primarily for the care of the elderly adult.

nursing, state board of   the department of state government that is responsible for administering the state nurse practice act. Some duties are testing applicants, licensing, registering and certifying, disciplining, and accrediting nursing education programs.

ombudsman   a person appointed by a governmental agency to hear and investigate complaints by private citizens against governmental agencies or officials. May also be an employee of a private agency, such as a health care facility.

opthalmologist   a physician who specializes in the problems of the eye.

optometrist   a specialist in the measurement of the powers of vision and the adaption of lenses or prisms for the aid of vision. Does not prescribe drugs.

osteoporosis   increased porosity of the bone, loss of denseness.

overt   open to view or knowledge, not concealed nor secret.

Parkinson's disease   a chronic nervous disease characterized by a fine, slowly spreading tremor, muscular weakness, rigidity, and a peculiar gait.

perineal   concerning or situated on the perineum.

perineum   the space between the vulva and the anus in the female, between the scrotum and the anus in the male.

phebothrombosis   the development of venous thrombi in the absence of associated inflammation.

pleura   serous membrane that enfolds the lungs and is reflected on the walls of the thorax and diaphragm.

pleural   containing the pleura (pl), a serous membrane containing the lungs and lining the walls of the thoracic cavity, the two layers enclosing a potential space, the pleural cavity.

pneumoencephalogram   a radiographic visualization of the fluid containing structures of the brain after cerebrospinal fluid is intermittently withdrawn by lumbar puncture and replaced by air, oxygen, or helium.

pneumonia   inflammation of the lungs with exudation and consolidation. **lobar p.**   an acute infectious disease due to the pneumococcus and marked by inflammation of one or more lobes of the lung. **hypostatic p.**   caused by constantly remaining in one position. Fluids become congested in one part of the lung. **aspiration p.**   due to aspiration of foreign material into the lungs.

podiatrist   chiropodist; a specialist in podiatry.

podiatry   chiropody, the specialty dealing with the study and care of the foot.

polypharmacy   1. administration of many drugs together. 2. administration of excessive medication.

postural drainage   drainage of secretions from the bronchi or a cavity in the lung by placing the patient's head lower than the area to be drained.

P.R.N.   Latin abbreviation *pro re nata*, as needed, as desired.

prognosis   a forecast of the probable course and outcome of a disorder.

proprietary   a privately owned business with profit as its objective.

Proteus   a genus of gram negative, mobile bacteria usually found in fecal and other putrefying matter.

psychic   concerning the mind or soul.

psychosis, senile   mental deterioration in old age with organic brain changes, the symptoms including impaired memory for recent events, irritability, etc.

rapport   a relationship of confidence and sympathy.

ritualism   the adherence to or insistence on ritual.

orthostatic hypotension   low blood pressure occurring when assuming an upright position after lying prone.

pulmonary infarction   a localized area of ischemic necrosis produced by occlusion of the pulmonary artery.

senescence   the process of growing old.

senile   pertaining to old age.

skilled care   a designation of DHEW for care of patients with complex needs. Requires professional nursing care 24 hours per day.

somatic   pertaining to or characteristic of the body.

staphylococcus   a genus of gram positive bacteria, constantly present on the skin and upper respiratory tract.

statutes   law, an enactment made by a legislature and written in a formal document.

stoma   a mouthlike opening, particularly a surgical opening for drainage or other purposes.

stroke   see *cerebro-vascular accident.*

subpoenaed   a legal writ requiring appearance in court to give testimony.

surrogate   a substitute; a thing or person that takes the place of something or someone else.

syncope   a faint, temporary loss of consciousness.

terminal   a termination, end, death.

thanatology   the science of death.

thrombophlebitis   a clot accompanied by inflammation of the affected vein.

thrombus   a solid mass formed in the living heart or vessels from the constituents of blood.

tomograph   an apparatus for moving the X-ray through an arc during an exposure, thus showing in detail a predetermined plane of tissue, while blurring details of other planes.

tomography   body section radiography by means of the tomograph.

trauma   a wound or injury, whether physical or psychic.

trochanter roll   a roll of material placed against the hip to maintain position and to prevent its outward rotation.

utilization review   an interdisciplinary committee that reviews the patient's need for care periodically based upon community care standards.

vertigo   sensation of rotation or movement; dizziness.

vibration   a shaking movement of the hands.

viral   pertaining to or caused by a virus.

vital capacity   the volume of air that can be expelled following full inspiration.

vulva   the external genital organs of the female, the mons pubis, labia majora and minora, clitoris, and vestibule of the vagina.

Answers to Review Questions

CHAPTER ONE

1. (a) Services needed by the elderly are inadequate in many parts of the United States because of the rapidly growing numbers of old people and the relative powerlessness of the elderly.

   (b) The elderly adult may find that due to negative stereotyping of the aged, he is denied some of the social and business contacts open to younger persons.

2. With the aid of a homemaker and meals-on-wheels, Mrs. Jones can return to her own home rather than being admitted to a long-term care facility.

3. When applying for a position in a long-term care facility, the practical nurse should ask:

   (a) What is the philosophy of the agency?

   (b) Are there written policies and procedures?

   (c) Are her skills and knowledge adequate for the description? Does the agency job description correlate with the legal description of practical nurses in her state?

(d) Is there provision for in-service education?

4. Institutionalization is the best approach for care of the elderly adult:

(a) when it is not safe for the patient to live by himself;

(b) when housing is inadequate;

(c) when the patient needs 24-hour nursing care;

(d) when diet or treatment is necessary that cannot be provided at home.

CHAPTER TWO

1. To survive to advanced years, it is necessary to:

(a) exercise regularly, remain active;

(b) keep weight normal, reduce animal-fat content of "normal" American diet;

(c) do not smoke or drink to excess and avoid air pollution;

(d) have long-lived ancestors.

2. To facilitate communication with the hard-of-hearing,

(a) raise voice only moderately, enunciate slowly and clearly;

(b) use written notes.

3. Sexual intercourse for the woman will be entirely possible. It may be uncomfortable at first, but adequate preparation will facilitate vaginal penetration. You cannot answer for the male partner as you have no information concerning his status.

4. The elderly are prone to respiratory problems because the lungs expand less and work less efficiently, coughing is less efficient, and circulation due to decreased activity is less.

5. No, intellect remains intact unless there is a disease process in the brain that results in reduced circulation and oxygenation. Some temporary clouding of the intellect may occur with serious systemic infections or other occurrances.

CHAPTER THREE

1. Crisis is that period when past problem-solving methods are not adequate to cope with the present situation. Examples are: (a)

death of a spouse, (b) retirement, (c) career change, and (d) societal attitudes.

2. In anxiety, the patient may become withdrawn or unnaturally talkative, or restless, with crying episodes; sleep and eating patterns may be disturbed.

3. Depression may result from hypoglycemia and may be caused by (a) meals too far apart, (b) meals containing excess carbohydrates and inadequate protein, (c) not enough food, or (d) need for supplementary feedings.

4. Suicide rates for elderly adults may be incorrect because they may use covert behavior such as (a) omission of necessary medications, (b) starvation, or (c) exposure, rather than violent acts.

5. The danger of suicide is the greatest when depression seems to improve; this may indicate that the patient is at peace because he has made his decision to die.

6. The acute brain syndrome is usually reversible if treated, as it has a physical basis such as myocardial infarction, pneumonia, hypoglycemia or hypocalemia, dehydration, mild stroke, or drug toxicity.

CHAPTER FOUR

1. It is important to have good rapport with the patient's family because:

   (a) it helps to reduce guilt feelings the family may have;

   (b) it helps decrease their fears and anxiety;

   (c) it helps the patient relax, feel trust, that his loved ones are treated with consideration.

2. Loss of privacy in the environment results in insecurity, loss of the sense of control of one's life, and feelings of loss of competency to cope with problems. Loss of privacy that exposes the body results in loss of self-respect and may cause humiliation.

3. (a) Do not dismiss the complaints.

   (b) Be sure there is no explainable reason for the complaint.

   (c) Give the patient extra attention, with plenty of touch.

4. The goal of diversional activities in a long-term care facility is to involve each resident in one or more activities that will assist in keeping him mentally, physically, and socially active.

5. The nurse may assist the bedfast patient by

   (a) providing a visit by a clergyman if the patient permits;

   (b) seeing that he is provided with the religious materials he needs;

   (c) reading to him, if necessary;

   (d) listening to his concerns.

CHAPTER FIVE

1. Some of the changes in life style that result from retirement are:

   (a) social contacts with coworkers are lost;

   (b) recreational outlets are lost;

   (c) income is reduced;

   (d) health care benefits are lost;

   (e) leisure time is abundant;

   (f) meaningful work is lost, prestige is reduced.

2. Leisure time can be made more useful by engaging in

   (a) interesting hobbies, particularly if they can be used to increase income;

   (b) further education;

   (c) service to others;

   (d) some travel.

3. The retiree should have supplemental insurance if he is not yet 65 and therefore not eligible for Medicare, or if his income is too high to receive Medicaid. Medicare does not cover all medical expenses.

4. The dying patient can be helped to feel he is not isolated

   (a) if he can remain in his customary room;

   (b) if he stays ambulatory as long as possible;

   (c) if the doors of his room are left open;

   (d) if visitors are encouraged.

5. In caring for a dying patient, some essential nursing care might be discontinued if

   (a) the care may cause severe pain;

(b) the care may be extremely tiring;

(c) the patient does not wish the care to be given, or the family requests that it be discontinued, or the doctor discontinues the order.

6. It is good practice to involve relatives in some aspects of terminal care because it makes death a reality and it helps the grief process and may shorten it.

CHAPTER SIX

1. Wasting not related to nerve damage can be reversed. This can be done by passive or active range of motion exercises, increased ambulation, good nutrition, and freedom from pain.

2. (a) Circulatory/statis—reverse by activity, passive and active exercises, tilt tables, and ambulation.

   (b) Eliminative disturbances—reverse by adding roughage to the diet and providing adequate toileting opportunities.

   (c) Urinary disturbances—reverse by increasing fluids, increasing activity, and toileting frequently.

   (d) Respiratory changes—reverse by frequent positional changes, deep breathing, coughing, and increasing activity.

3. Pressure sores usually occur on bony prominences such as the sacrum, shoulder blade, ischial tuberosities, elbows, heels, and trochanters. Early symptoms of decubiti include redness and indentations in skin, blebs, and occasionally skin darkening.

4. Some causes of decubiti are pressure, trauma, lack of circulation, poor nutritional level, low hemoglobin, prolonged wetting by urine, feces, or perspiration.

5. For oral care of the unconscious patient:

   (a) use a dry brush, gauze, or dry terry facecloth to prevent aspiration;

   (b) stimulate the gums by massage;

   (c) clean the tongue and lubricate the lips;

   (d) use a moistening agent in the mouth;

6. Good grooming promotes comfort and self-esteem and makes the patient more acceptable to family and friends.

CHAPTER SEVEN

1. Special safety precautions are necessary because more elderly patients:

    (a) have poor vision;

    (b) have slow reaction time;

    (c) may be weak or confused;

    (d) have arthritic changes;

    (e) are more prone to side effects from medication.

2. Before restraints are applied, the following steps should be taken:

    (a) assess the patient for any trauma;

    (b) take vital signs to identify any physical changes;

    (c) review the list of medications to attempt to identify untoward drug reactions;

    (d) attempt to find causes of agitation;

    (e) if necessary, call physician to report patient's condition and ask for permission to use restraints if other nursing measures have failed.

3. After restraints are applied,

    (a) be sure restraints are not impairing circulation;

    (b) turn the patient frequently;

    (c) ambulate, if possible;

    (d) sit up in bed;

    (e) remove restraints and massage limbs frequently;

    (f) be sure restraints are applied so that the patient cannot loosen or remove;

    (g) observe the patient frequently.

4. The nurse has greater responsibilities for medications in a long-term care facility than in an acute care area because:

    (a) there is no pharmacist in the building;

    (b) patients are not seen daily by the physician;

    (c) patients are taking more drugs;

    (d) individual reactions to drugs are different in elderly adults.

5. Some hazards you might encounter with dangerous substances in a nursing facility are:

(a) unattended, unlocked drug carts or trays;

(b) patent medicines in bedside drawers;

(c) cleaning materials on housekeepers' carts;

(d) antiseptics or other chemicals in unlocked utility rooms.

6. The following changes in the body of the elderly adult affect the results of medications:

(a) body weight and fluid are reduced;

(b) cardiac reserve and output are reduced;

(c) venous congestion increases;

(d) oxygen adsorption and exchange are reduced;

(e) kidney and liver function are reduced.

CHAPTER EIGHT

1. Changes in diet are difficult to maintain because of peoples' past memories of food, their religion, ethnic background, and past habits of eating.

2. If carbohydrates are missing from the diet, the body will use protein for energy rather than for body repair and maintenance.

3. The following problems might face the elderly person who is trying to provide himself an adequate diet:

(a) inadequate diet knowledge;

(b) insufficient income for food;

(c) inadequate transportation to markets;

(d) lack of cooking area;

(e) physical inability to cook or shop;

(f) no knowledge of or experience in cooking.

4. Calories should be reduced in the diet of the elderly adult because of:

(a) lower activity levels;

(b) lower cellular activity;

(c) lower basal metabolism.

5. Limitation of sodium will allow the body to remove fluid by diuresis, which will reduce the labor of the heart.

6. A diet lower in animal fat content is indicated for the person with atherosclerosis.

7. If a patient must be fed, the following actions by the nurse will help to assure that the patient has a pleasant mealtime:

   (a) complete personal hygiene measures;

   (b) arrange room in an orderly manner;

   (c) have food within sight of the patient;

   (d) have the patient sitting up in bed;

   (e) allow the patient to participate in feeding as much as possible.

CHAPTER NINE

1. Pulse rates rise because:

   (a) cardiac output decreases;

   (b) stroke volume decreases;

   (c) pulse rate increases to assure constant cardiac output.

2. If the patient's blood pressure is 165/100 upon admission, it is above the norm and needs treatment and/or medication. It should be reported to the charge nurse or physician.

3. It is difficult for the elderly adult to maintain homeostasis because the defense mechanisms of the body have become less efficient and do not react quickly, and strength and energy may be decreased.

4. It is important to establish and maintain a data base of the patient's vital signs and weight in order to have a reliable measurement with which to compare new data; normal measurements may be elevated ones for this patient.

5. In the elderly adult, changes in the immune system result in slow and/or ineffective reaction to antibodies.

Index